Focused Problem Resolution

# Focused
# Problem
# Resolution

## Selected Papers of the
## MRI Brief Therapy Center

*Edited by*
**Richard Fisch, MD**
**Wendel A. Ray, PhD**
*and*
**Karin Schlanger, LMFT**

**ZEIG, TUCKER & THEISEN, INC.**

Phoenix  Arizona

**Library of Congress Cataloging-in-Publication Data**

Focused problem resolution: Selected papers of the MRI brief therapy / Ray, Wendel A. — 1st
edition.
   p.      cm.

   Includes bibliographic references.
   ISBN   978-1-9324442-35-7  (alk. paper)
   1. Brief psychotherapy.        2. Counseling — mental health
   3. Family — Psychological aspects.
   I. Ray, Wendel      II. Title

616.89'14 — dc21

Published by

Zeig, Tucker & Theisen, Inc.
3618 North 24th Street
Phoenix, AZ 85016

Manufactured in the United States of America

# Contents

# Acknowledgements

Completion of this volume—the placement of published and unpublished papers, recordings and other artifacts from researchers at the MRI Brief Therapy Center into a computer data base, and editing of the manuscript—is, in large part, a product of the hard work over the years of able graduate assistants from the Marriage and Family Therapy Doctoral and Master Degree Programs at the University of Louisiana at Monroe: John Miller, David Govener, Craig Moorman, Jana Sutton, Pearl Wong, Cary Brown, Molly Govener, Matthew Boer, Ryan Stivers, and especially Courtney Brasher whose amazing proofreading skills are gratefully acknowledged. Many of these individuals have long since graduated and are teaching and serving in positions of leadership in the field of systemic marriage and family therapy.

The chapters in this book have been previously published in the publications noted in the footnotes printed at the bottom of the first page of each chapter. Copyright resides with these publications, and grateful acknowledgement is expressed for permission to reprint these papers in this book.

New material in these volumes include the "Introduction" by Richard Fisch, M.D., (pp. ix-xiii), and "One thing leads to another," redux (pp. xiv-xxv) by Wendel A. Ray, Ph.D. and Karin Schlanger, LMFT which are copyright © 2009 by Zeig, Tucker, Theisan and Company, Limited, the publisher of this work. All rights reserved. Permission to reproduce any part of this work in any form must be obtained in writing from the copyright holder.

# Introduction[1]

## Richard Fisch, M.D.

The idea and planning of a clinical research project in brief therapy began at MRI in 1965. The climate of therapy at that time had reached the highpoint of psychoanalysis and it, or variations of it, influenced much, if not most of therapy activity. At the same time, family therapy was beginning to develop but had very little recognition in the therapy world. As with many new developments, adherents to it found new features to embellish its practices: including the family pet in sessions, requiring that all sessions address the entire nuclear family, occasionally conducting sessions in the family home, exploring past influence by the families of origin on the current family members as children and including, in an occasional session, individuals who had any ongoing contact with the family (such as the local mail carrier, a store keeper, local police officer, children's teachers among other people. Therapists who practiced this technique might have 30 or 40 people in the session.)

As one can tell, these embellishments resulted in more time spent in conducting the therapy. When family therapy was first developed and introduced it was seen as a method for resolving problems much more rapidly than traditional therapies. With the lengthening of therapy, it began to approximate time spent in those traditional approaches, time measured in years rather than months or, certainly, weeks.

It was in that climate that the Brief Therapy Center was formed. Much of the impetus for it came from our awareness of novel methods of others which enhanced brevity of treatment. Principle among them was Milton Erickson, a

---

[1] Parts of this introduction are reprinted from the introduction to R. Fisch & W. Ray (Guest editors), (2005). Principles of problem formation & problem resolution, 39 years of innovation at the Mental Research Institute Brief Therapy Center, a special double issue on the MRI Approach, *Journal of Brief Therapy*, 4, (1 & 2).

psychiatrist and Jay Haley, an associate in the Bateson project and member of MRI. While each differed in their styles and methods of conducting therapy, there was a considerable overlap. For example, their emphasis was on prescribing some activity for the client(s) to be carried out between sessions. "Insight" was either a small factor in the overall treatment or was used to legitimize the prescribed intervention. This latter feature was likely considered necessary since the suggestions offered ran counter to what might be called "common sense." Thus, to the average person, client or visiting therapist, these directives seemed strange, "off the wall" or "paradoxical." Our group found them puzzling yet intriguing especially since they were able to bring about desired change rather rapidly.

We spent several months discussing and organizing our research methodology. Our initial model was very broad and vague: to develop an approach to therapy which would be "effective" yet "brief." On that basis we gave the project the name of "Brief Therapy Center" (a title we later came to regret as we will explain later in this introduction.) We readily agreed that we would set a session limit to every case. At first, one of us said "How about 20 sessions?" However, since that could cover 6 months of treatment "it didn't seem brief," and so we quickly decided that 10 sessions sounded sufficiently brief. We also quickly decided we would see whomever sought help and not filter out clients because of the nature of their problems or "diagnosis." Related to that, we decided that rather than pair clients to a particular therapist (because of a special talent or experience) client/therapist matching would be randomized. At first, we planned on setting a few hours a week for the whole group to discuss and aid in planning the primary therapist's treatment; also that the therapist would bring in his clinical notes to aid in that discussion. At that suggestion, there was a wild moan (scream?) from the rest of us since we didn't want to wait for days to find out what was happening in the therapy. Since MRI had already had a one-way mirror with an observation room, we decided we would all observe our compatriot during his therapy and then discuss that after the session was over. (Several years later we were surprised—and amused—to learn that visitors to our project had begun setting up one-way mirror observation in their own work setting believing that it was an integral part of our model. For us, it was done (initially) only because of our impatience although later we found it to be useful as well as having drawbacks.)

We wisely decided not to begin seeing clients until we had formulated a method for evaluating the outcome of the therapy. While all other elements in our methodology took only a few weeks, on this item we spent about three months. We considered and then rejected almost all of the standard methods. (One of us suggested we only treat obese patients and their families because then we could "easily measure change by seeing how much they weighed at the end of treatment." That colleague was not put off when we said that since we look at problems from an interactional point (of view), rather than an individual one, weighing one member would not be conclusive since another member of the family might have gained weight. He immediately replied that would be no problem since we could rent a freight scale and weigh the whole family.)

Finally, one of us and this author does not remember who, said "a client comes in because he/she has a problem. If we are to assess any change for which our therapy was instrumental, then at the termination of treatment the client shouldn't have the problem." We all believed this simple, straightforward and sensible approach would be appropriate for our purpose and this formed the basis for our follow-up practice.

With that out of the way, we began. Our beginnings might best be described as earnest, thoughtful and friendly chaos. To begin with, our professional backgrounds were a mélange of different psychoanalytic schools. (The author's was a mixture of traditional Freudian analysis coupled with a Sullivanian twist, John Weakland's mostly Freudian and Paul Watzlawick's Jungian. We had all used Ericksonian hypnosis in our practices and at same time, we had all incorporated notions and practices of family therapy.)

Early in our planning we had assumed that one element of outcome would be to delineate patients for whom brief therapy was suitable from those for whom it was not. This assumption changed very early in our work, some of the change coming from our decision to use the same limit of sessions with every patient. Some of it came from our own experience of success with patients when we had "experimented" with some techniques used by Erickson and Haley which gave us the bias that it can work. Thus our thinking of outcome shifted to see how much, with any case, can be achieved within a ten session limit. A little later this optimistic bent influenced our procedure in the follow-up evaluation. Originally we thought of assessing only problem change. We decided to add two other elements for study:

1. When there has been a successful change in the primary problem, is there the development of new problems? (a variant of the psychoanalytic idea of "symptom substitution")
2. The corollary: when the primary problem has been resolved, is there *improvement* in any other problems the patient had alluded to during treatment but for which no attempt was made to resolve it? (Over the years, outcome reports showed extremely little new problems (< 1%) but significant improvement in "untouched" problems (25 %).)

Other changes in our thinking and strategies developed as we stumbled our way while working with patients. Probably the most strategic change occurred when we began to notice that, with little exception, clients seemed to be very "naïve" in their attempts to resolve or deal with their problem. This led to an unexpected but strategic change in our clinical approach. We were working with a man coming in about his very young son who was terrified about starting school. His reaction to being urged to go to school was so pitiful that his parents usually found some excuse to let him stay home. On the rare instance that he would allow himself to be taken to school, this "success" was short lived since the school nurse would call the home explaining that their son was so upset she felt it necessary they come to school and take him home. The child never completed one day of school. At the time we felt that the child's fear was a manifestation of a marital conflict between the parents and we were planning to gear our treatment strategy toward that focus. However, we thought it would enhance that effort if first we could influence the father to be less "naïve" about his son's fear of school. In his efforts to ease the child's fear, he had tried to reassure him about school: "I met your teacher and she is a kind friendly person." "When I was starting school I found it was fun and enjoyed it a lot." Instead, we asked him to tell the child that he hadn't been quite truthful about his own school experience and that he had actually been quite frightened. He agreed and at the next appointment two weeks later, he said he had done that. We were about to ask to see his wife (In preparation for marital therapy) when he announced that his son was now going to school every day and without any urging from him.

In effect, it was the first case where we developed the idea that the problem had more to do with the father's way of attempting to resolve the child's fear than any other explanation. Success with a new effort tends to encourage repetition and so we began to ask clients how they had attempted to resolve or alleviate the problem they were coming in about, what we later called their "attempted solution." With subsequent success we made "the attempted solution" and its departure by the client the bedrock of our model.

Space for this introductory section does not permit describing fully all of the measures we developed in refining the therapy: the use of implicit optimism to achieve or enhance change in the problem, varieties of prescribed interventions, the careful use of language and semantics, among other procedures. Our efforts with clients and the underlying simplicity of our model enabling success in "clinical" cases later tempted us to use that same model in "non-clinical" problems: business and corporate problems, school problems, dealing with a speeding violation, and reducing conflict in a broad variety of interpersonal problems of everyday life. And these experiences lead to the comment early in this introduction of why we regret the name of "Brief Therapy Center."

First of all, "brief" is too loose a term to make much sense. It's like those labels on food products describing the contents as "light," "low calorie," "popular," and the like. (Whenever people hear about "brief therapy" they ask "How brief is brief therapy?" How come they never ask "How long is long-term therapy?" Also, "therapy" implies "clinical" work in which the clients have some special type of problem: mental, psychological, neurotic, nervous breakdowns...(take your pick). We finally realized that "clinical" and "non-clinical" were unnecessary and limiting separations for doing the same thing, helping to resolve human interpersonal problems. In that sense we don't do "therapy" but problem solving. Unavoidably, "Interpersonal Problem Solving Center" does not have the cachet that "Brief Therapy Center" has.

# "One Thing Leads to Another," *Redux*[2]

## *Wendel A. Ray* and *Karin Schlanger*

> "Though I find [Dick Fisch, John Weakland, and
> Paul Watzlawick] different persons, when they
> are working or talking professionally I feel the
> presence of Don Jackson hovering above them
> and Gregory Bateson off in the distance"
> —Andrew Ferber (1972, p. 32).

The Mental Research Institute (MRI) has a distinguished history and can lay claim as the birthplace of numerous contributions to Communication/Interactional theory and innovations in the application of these ideas in the practice of family and brief therapy—not least of which is to be home of the MRI Brief Therapy Center (BTC). When Richard Fisch, M.D., proposed to Don Jackson the creation at MRI of a "Brief Therapy Clinic and Evaluation Project" (Fisch, 1965a) no comparable research endeavor had ever been undertaken. Jackson "was a developer of brief therapy when long-term therapy was the fashion" (Haley, 2005). The creation of this Center launched a new way of doing therapy: brief therapy. Since the BTC was founded many other forms of brief therapy have emerged in the field, and we would like to take this opportunity, in keeping with what we currently practice at MRI, to describe the BTC model of problem-solving brief therapy.

Inspired by the clinical work of Milton Erickson, Don Jackson (1961), and Jay Haley (1963), Fisch envisioned a research center determined to break away

---

[2] This title is borrowed from, and in honor of, an earlier paper published by John Weakland describing his recollections of the Gregory Bateson Research Projects. See Weakland, J. (1981). One thing leads to another, In C. Wilder & J.Weakland (Eds.) *Rigor and Imagination – Essays from the legacy of Gregory Bateson.* New York: Praeger, p. 43-64.

from what was then an almost exclusively individual and pathology orientation that dominated psychotherapy. Following in the tradition of the Bateson Research Project (Bateson, Jackson, Haley & Weakland, 1956, 1963), Fisch and colleagues sought to create "a clinic not organized toward pathology but toward the reconstitutive processes of human beings" (Jackson, 1965a), which explicitly focused on making therapy more effective and efficient. Funding was secured (Jackson, 1965b, 1966 a, b, & c), a clinic established, operating procedures developed, and in early January 1967 researchers at the BTC began seeing clients.

In the forty-three years since the Brief Therapy Center was created Fisch, Weakland, Watzlawick and colleagues have conducted thousands of hours of therapy, published more than forty books, hundreds of journal articles and book chapters, and trained legions of mental health professionals from all over the world in MRI Brief Therapy.

Dick Fisch delights in demythologizing the innovations introduced at the BTC, but one wonders what the state of clinical practice would be today were it not for the theoretical and practice innovations introduced at the BTC. Conceptual and intervention strategies and procedures pioneered at the BTC have been adopted by most other models of practice and training—so extensively used that who it was that introduced them has become obscured with the passage of time—

- Routine use of therapy teams,
- Recording of all sessions, first by audio then video once the technology allowed, to encourage transactional analysis and to enhance effectiveness,
- Use of the one-way viewing screen, the telephone and in-session breaks for consultation with the team of observers,
- Setting a limit on the number of sessions (ten in the case of the BTC, with an actual average of 6 ½ [see chapter 18]), to encourage accountability (on the part of client and therapist alike),

—are all innovations established at the BTC that are now so widely accepted practices in training institutes that it is easy to forget that their use must have started somewhere—there was—the MRI Brief Therapy Center.

Willingness to question what Weakland termed the *received wisdom* (long held and unquestioned assumptions about behavior and clinical procedures), and to let go of ideas when not useful in the actual practice of therapy, are standard protocols at the BTC, where the search for more effective and efficient techniques for helping people change created an atmosphere of creativity and experimentation from which countless clinical innovations emerged.

Researchers at the BTC were and remain intent on demystifying the practice of effective therapy and Fisch, Weakland, Watzlawick and colleagues devoted more than four decades to spelling out *how to do* therapy effectively.

To adequately describe the multitude of ways the BTC has shaped present day clinical intervention requires much more space than this introduction allows for, so only a few will be highlighted.

- The BTC Team took observable transactions taking place in the here and now between members of the clients' relationship nexus *and* between the client and therapist as the base-line data for understanding behavior. Inferences about historic traumatic experiences, genetic, or biochemical causes were relevant only in terms of understanding the client's frame of reference and explanatory stance. Primary focus is on how problems are called forth, maintained and perpetuated in interactions taking place the clients real life (see Chapter 1, 3, 5, and 7).
- Realization of the vital importance of discerning who is the person most motivated in a family or other interactional nexus willing and able to change. Most of the therapeutic work is then done with that person (see chapter 6 and 12).
- Experimenting with various methods of persuasion to influence clients to take action that is different from what they have tried until now (i.e. to desist from problem maintaining behavior) (see chapter 8 and 9).
- Recognizing and writing about the now commonplace idea that how one goes about motivating someone requires knowing who it is you are trying to motivate. This obvious but profound idea—now routinely accepted in the therapy world—that helping people change requires inquiring into and learning the client's world view, frame of reference, and situational / contextual circumstances—what the BTC term *client position*—is basic to effective problem-solving brief therapy (see chapter 3, 14 and 16).
- Adopting an uncompromising *non-pathological, non-normative* way on the part of the therapist to view and engage the client (see chapter 2 and 16).
- Knowing when, how, and with whom to inquire to make plain the problem as clearly and specifically as possible in concrete terms, (i.e., for whom the problem is a problem, in what way it is a problem). Weakland often said that the first step of effective brief treatment requires obtaining a clear, behavioral description of the problem *before* inquiring into efforts being made to solve the problem (i.e. attempted solutions) (see chapter 4 and 18).
- From the BTC perspective, the solution is the problem; interrupt the solution behavior that maintains and perpetuates the problem and the problem virtually always goes away with no further intervention re-

quired. Inquiring into ineffective attempted solutions (i.e. what unwitting behaviors function to maintain or reinforce the problem) is the second step in the approach. Dr. Fisch often says effective brief therapy interrupts problem maintaining attempted solutions more than actual problems. (see chapter 9, 13, and 14).

* Emphasis is placed on sticking with observable, concrete behavior, _and_ discerning the client's explanatory frame to aid in framing suggestions in ways that are consonant with the client's position (see chapter 6).
* Placing importance on _indirectly_ influencing the client to _act differently_, as in contrast to trying to promote change by evoking insight, is a key to efficient and effective problem resolution (see chapter 17 and 18).

Fisch, Weakland, Watzlawick and colleagues focused on developing coherent, consistent, effective, _learnable_ and _teachable_ skills in promoting constructive change, and in so doing created a time proven basic framework for effectively treating the widest range of emotional and behavioral problems. The BTC model of brief therapy became one of the most influential, some believe the most effective, treatment approaches in the field of brief therapy today (Fisch, Weakland & Segal, 1982; Fisch & Schlanger, 1999; Fisch & Ray, 2005; Ray & Watzlawick, 2005; Schlanger and Anger-Díaz, 2005; Schlanger and Martin, 1998; Herr & Weakland, 1979; Nardone & Watzlawick, 1993; Watzlawick, Beavin-Bavelas, & Jackson, 1967; Watzlawick, Weakland, & Fisch, 1974; Watzlawick & Weakland, 1977; Watzlawick, 1976; Weakland, Fisch, Watzlawick, & Bodin, 1974; Weakland & Ray, 1995).

The MRI Brief Therapy conception of problem formation and problem resolution is elegant in its simplicity:

* It is less the problem itself, but the efforts being made to solve it that inadvertently perpetuate and exacerbate the problem.
* Successfully interrupt the unsuccessful attempted solutions and the problem usually dissipates without need for further intervention.

As apparently simple as is this framework, the _practice_ of therapy based on this conception to problem formation and problem resolution is not as easy as it sounds.

The BTC approach is grounded in more than sixty years of research that intentionally _does not rely_ on conventional, individually oriented theories of human behavior. Rather, the MRI Brief Therapy model derives from the work of Gregory Bateson, Milton Erickson, and Don D. Jackson. The model focuses on making sense of complaints and symptomatic behavior in terms of how it fits within the relational contexts (family and social) of which it is a part. The "data" of the orientation is **actual behavior** of the complainant and those with whom he/she interacts. *How* is the problem behavior a problem, in *what way* is it a problem, and *to whom* is it a problem described in concrete behavioral terms? The model of causality used to comprehend complaints or problems is *cybernetic*—that is understanding and explaining all behavior in terms of its place in a wider, ongoing, organized system of behavior involving feedback and recursive reinforcement (see chapter 1 and 16). Problem behavior is understood **not** in terms of deficits or abnormality, but rather as adaptive within the broader context (see chapter 3, 7, 10 and 13).

The model of brief therapy pioneered by Fisch, Weakland, and Watzlawick is explicitly a *strategic* orientation (see chapter 6, and Fisch, Weakland & Segal, 1982) that seeks to promote the *minimum change* required to resolve the presenting problem, rather than trying to restructure the whole family system. To reiterate, conceptually the MRI brief therapy model is quite simple—a problem can persist only if efforts to solve it are ineffective. Once clear understanding of the problem is achieved, primary attention is given to how people themselves and other around them are attempting to solve the problem, because the problem is inadvertently maintained and perpetuated by ineffective efforts to solve it. When the clients' efforts to solve the problem are successfully interrupted, the problem quickly resolves itself.

As one of, if not the first, social constructivist orientations (see chapter 15, 17, and Watzlawick 1976, 1978, and 1984), MRI Brief Therapy takes seriously the second order cybernetic position that ideas and premises the therapist holds about the nature of problems and treatment strongly influence what is focused on, whom is seen in treatment, what is said and done; and equally, what is not said and done when working with the client. The therapists' presuppositions can facilitate change *or* contribute to maintenance of the problem. *Transparency*, congruency between theory and practice, and outcome —i.e. *effectiveness* of therapy—are the measures used by BTC researchers to shape the evolution of the approach:

> … our theory is just a conceptual map of our approach to understanding and treating the kinds of problems therapists meet in daily practice. Like any map, it is basically a tool to help someone find his way from one place to another—in this case from the therapists encountering a client's problem to its successful resolution. As a tool, a map is never the actuality, is always provisional, and is to be judged primarily by the results of its use…
> Just as one cannot *not* communicate, since in a social setting even silence is a message, one cannot *not* theorize. We aim to make our fundamental views—our premises and assumptions—as explicit as possible, since the other danger for theory arises when it is inexplicit. We all have

general ideas which form the context for, and thus guide, our specific thinking and behavior. These may be implicit and taken for granted. Then they are all the more influential, since they are less open to review, questioning, and possible revision. ... Therefore, we attempt to make our premises and assumptions, and their relationship to our practices as clear and explicit as possible (Fisch, Weakland, & Segal, 1982, p. 7).

## Case Example

An example may further clarify the basic orientation. A 32-year-old mother initiated therapy because she was afraid of her 15-year-old daughter. In a recent tirade the daughter broke all the windows in the house, had threatened to kill her mother, then tried to cut her own arm off with a rusty machete. Angry and exhausted, the mother was threatening to send the girl to a state school. The mother's main attempt to handle the daughter's outbursts involved reasoning with her, to which the girl would respond with escalating verbal abuse and threats, followed by the mother trying to appear "in control" and not show how upset she was.

In therapy the mother was convinced to refrain from "reasoning with an unreasonable person," and instead consider what she might else do, something perhaps uncharacteristic of her usual approach. The mother said she could stop trying to look calm and in control and instead show her daughter how afraid she was for her future. The mother implemented the suggestion with almost immediate positive results. The next day when her daughter threw a tantrum while riding the car, the mother pulled over, parked, and broke down crying in despair over her fear that her daughter would come to a bad end if she continued to be "out of control." The daughter tried to calm and reassure her mother, who cried uncontrollably until her daughter was able to help her calm down by calming down herself and apologizing for her outburst. As the mother successfully avoided reasoning (the central theme of her past attempted solution), the daughter exhibited fewer and less dramatic temper tantrums. With the daughter's behavior much improved and the problem resolved to the satisfaction of the mother and daughter, after four sessions therapy was concluded. At one year follow-up the clients reported continued resolution of the problem.

**Question?** I've been familiar with the MRI Brief Therapy approach for a long time. Could you describe ways the models have evolved in recent years?

There have been many refinements, two of which will be highlighted: First, great emphasis is placed on listening closely to what the client says. In contrast to many approaches that emphasize the importance of listening for the underlying meaning embedded in what a client says, MRI Brief Therapists do the opposite of that. We listen closely to exactly what the client is saying and how they are saying it. This not only conveys respect, but it helps the therapist understand how the client thinks and feels about the problem. This is called getting the clients *position* in the MRI Brief Therapy approach and is vital to understanding how to respond to the client in ways that utilize his or her language and world view, and in so doing accessing the cooperation of the client in efforts to resolve the problem.

A second important advancement is the intentional use of implication. As the nuances of human interaction have become clearer, so has the vital importance of avoiding the intentional or unintentional placing of blame on the client or any of his or her important others. The evoking of blame is the same as rejecting the client, can increase defensiveness, and make eliciting the client's cooperation more difficult. To avoid these complications the intentional use of indirect messages on the part of the therapist has evolved as an important aspect of these models. Thus, embracing and investigating the notion that **what is implied** by what the therapist says is as influential, and in a sense more influential, than what is said explicitly. Thus close attention to the use of implication has become one of the important techniques used to promote productive change.

**Question?** With what kind of problems are appropriate to use MRI Brief Therapy with, and what is the success rate?

MRI Brief Therapy has demonstrated effectiveness in working with the widest range of difficult clinical problems, such as chronic mental illness, adolescent acting out, marital conflict, alcohol and substance abuse, family violence, depression, severe emotional problems, and psychosomatic disorders such as anorexia, bulimia, and ulcerated colitis. Outcome studies have demonstrated a success rate of 72% in early studies (Weakland, Fisch, Watzlawick, & Bodin, 1974) to 96% or higher rate of success in more recent studies (Chubb, 1995; Nardone, 1995). Work in the Latino Brief Therapy Center has demonstrated particular effectiveness in working with minority cultures. We believe this is the case, in part, because of the inherent respect for the client and their value system that this model ascribes to (Díaz, Schlanger, Rincon, & Mendoza, 2004). There a number of other domains beyond therapy for which MRI Brief Therapy has demonstrated effectiveness including administration, management, business consulting (Feinberg, 2007; Gill, 1999) and animal abuse (Loar, 1998) to name but a few.

This book brings together in one place a selection of the very best papers from the MRI Brief Therapy Center. Selecting papers for inclusion in this collection was not easy. Combined, Fisch, Weakland, Watzlawick published more than 250 articles and book chapters, and when contributions of other BTC associates were considered the number grew to more than 400. Fortunately, two collections of Watzlawick's papers have already been published (Watzlawick, 1989; Ray & Nardone, 2009), allowing focus of this volume to be on the most important papers written by John Weakland and Richard Fisch. Two of the most important pioneers of communication/interactional theory and brief therapy, Dick Fisch and John Weakland are our mentors to whom we owe a tremendous debt of gratitude for teaching us how to think and act in the practice of brief therapy, and in life in general.

Presented chronologically, the papers span nearly fifty years. In Chapter One, *Resistance to Change in the Psychiatric Community*, Dr. Fisch lucidly outlines resistances on the part of pathology oriented medical clinicians to a non-pathological, non-normative orientation.

Insightful and humorous, readers will enjoy Chapter Two, *On Unbecoming Family Therapists*, by Fisch, Weakland, Watzlawick, and Bodin which is the earliest published articulation of the MRI Brief Therapy orientation. In Chapter Three, *"The Double-Bind Theory" by Self-Reflexive Hindsight*, John Weakland reflects on the current relevance of the major contributions he and other Bateson Team members made to creation of communication theory. Chapter Four, *Brief Therapy: Focused Problem Resolution*, by Weakland, Fisch, Watzlawick, and Bodin, is the paper that launched the field of brief therapy. Published in 1974, this stunningly clear paper describes the logic and practices of MRI Brief Therapy, and reports the results of the first 100 clients seen at the BTC, thus providing the earliest outcome study in the emerging field of brief therapy. In Chapter Five, *Communication Theory and Clinical Change*, Weakland presents another classic articulation of the premises and practices of MRI Brief Therapy. Weakland and Fisch collaborate in Chapter Six, *The Strategic Approach*, to outline salient aspects of brief therapy as they emerge in the on-going research of the BTC Team.

In the ground-breaking Chapter Seven, *Family Somatics*, John Weakland focuses the application of principals of communication theory to medical illnesses. In Chapter Eight, *"Sometimes It's Better for the Right Hand Not to Know What the Left Hand is Doing,"* Fisch presents a fascinating full length case study of an adolescent with a congenitally disfigured hand and his parents in which the nuances of the model, especially the gentle art of reframing, are outlined. Chapter Nine, *OK—You've been a Bad Mother*, is an equally informative full case study by John Weakland in which the nuances of the successful practce of MRI Brief Therapy is revealed in dramatic form. Chapter Ten, *Pursuing the Evident into Schizophrenia & Beyond*, and Eleven, *The Double-Bind Theory: Some Current Implications for Child Psychiatry*, both by John Weakland, are among the clearest articulations extant of the relevance premises of communication theory to understanding behavior and how to promote constructive change.

In another ground-breaking article, Chapter Twelve, *Family Therapy with*

*Individuals*, Weakland contends that working from an interactional or systemic perspective has more to do with how the therapist conceptualizes problems than anything else, and very little to do with the number of people seen in therapy. The next chapter, *The Brief Treatment of Alcoholism*, by Fisch, offers a clear and compelling case study of successful therapy with an "alcoholic" woman by the uncompromising adherence to principles of MRI Brief Therapy. In Chapter Fourteen, *Cases that Don't Make Sense: Brief Strategic Treatment in Medical Practice*, Weakland and Fisch apply tenets of brief therapy to demystify and succeed in working with baffling medical complaints. The title of Chapter Fifteen, *Myths about Brief Therapy; Myths of Brief Therapy*, offers a tantalizing summary of Weakland's treatise, which addresses some of the misconceptions that have emerged in recent years as brief therapy has become popular. This is followed by another clear distillation by Fisch of fundamental premises and practices of the model in Chapter Sixteen, *Basic Elements in the Brief Therapies*. Dr. Fisch then turns his attention to addressing challenges made in the literature about the ethics of brief therapy in Chapter Seventeen, *To Thine Own Self be True—Ethical Issues in Strategic Therapy*. Published nearly thirty years after the BTC was founded, in Chapter Eighteen, *Brief Therapy—MRI Style*, Weakland and Fisch offers a report of advances made in the practice of Brief Therapy.

## Concluding Remarks

It is ironic that currently the Communication/Interactional Theory set forth by Gregory Bateson's Research Team, operationalized at the Mental Research Institute under Don Jackson's leadership, then refined during the past forty-three years by researchers in the Brief Therapy Center seems to be much more pervasively embraced across Europe and among Spanish speaking countries, Japanese, and other cultures around the globe than it is here in the United States. Indeed, to paraphrase Paul Watzlawick, the fame of the MRI Brief Therapy Center is inverse to the distance traveled from Palo Alto. In recent years both authors have even had the experience at conferences of people walking up and saying that while they had been influenced by the work of researchers at MRI and the BTC, with "advances" in genetic research and pharmaceutical intervention on the one hand, and the currently popular postmodern and language based models of practice on the other, they thought the Institute had long ago settled under the waters of obscurity.

Yet, to echo the sentiments of Mark Twain, reports of our demise have been greatly exaggerated. The basic premises of Interactional/Communication Theory remain salient, and MRI Brief Therapy remains among the most effective and efficient treatment approaches. The MRI Brief Therapy Center is alive and well, and increasing the reach of Brief Therapy through the Latino Brief

Therapy Center.

## References

Bateson, G., Jackson, D., Haley, J., & Weakland, J. (1956), Toward a theory of schizophrenia, *Behavioral Science*, 1 (4), 251-264.

Bateson, G., Jackson, D., Haley, J., & Weakland, J. (1963). A note on the double-bind—1962. *Family Process*, 2, (1), 154-161.

Cecchin, G., Lane, G., Ray, W. (1992). *Irreverence*, London, UK: Karnac.

Chubb. H. (1995). Outpatient clinic effectiveness with the MRI Brief Therapy Model. In J. Weakland & W. Ray (Eds.). *Propagations, Thirty Years of Influence from the Mental Research Institute*, pp. 129-132. New York: Haworth.

Díaz, B., Schlanger, K., Rincon, C., & Mendoze, A. (2004). Problem-solving across cultures: Our Latino Experience, *Journal of Systemic Therapies*, 23 (4), Winter, 28-28.

Feinberg, S. (2007). *The Advantage Makers*, Upper Saddle River, NJ: Pearson Educational, Inc.

Ferber, A., Mendelsohn, M., & Napier, A. (1972). *The Book of Family Therapy*. New York: Science House, p. 32.

Fisch, R. (1965). Memorandum dated September 15, 1965 to Don Jackson titled, *Proposal for Brief Therapy Clinic and Evaluation project*.

Fisch, R., Weakland, J., Segal, L. (1982). *The Tactics of Change—Doing Therapy Briefly*, San Francisco, CA: Jossey-Bass.

Fisch, R., & Schlanger, K. (1999). *Brief Therapy with Intimidating Cases—Changing the Unchangeable,* San Francisco, CA: Jossey-Bass.

Fisch, R., & Ray, W. (Eds.), (2005). Special double issue devoted to the MRI approach, *Journal of Brief Therapy*, 4, (1 & 2), 1-122.

Gill, L. (1999). *How to Work with Just About Anyone*, New York: Fireside.

Haley, J. (1963). *Strategies of Psychotherapy*, New York: Grune & Stratton, Inc.

Herr, J., & Weakland, J. (1989). *Counseling with Elders and their Families*, New York: Springer.

Jackson, D. (1961). Interactional Psychotherapy. In W. Ray, (Ed.), (2009). *Don D. Jackson, M.D., Interactional Theory in Clinical Practice, Selected Papers Vol. II*, Phoenix, AZ: Zeig, Tucker, Theisan, Ltd.

Jackson, D. (Ed.), (1968a). *Communication, Family & Marriage: Human Communication, Volume I*, Palo Alto, CA: Science & Behavior Books.

Jackson, D. (Ed.), (1968b). *Communication, Therapy and Change: Human Communication, Volume II*, Palo Alto, CA: Science & Behavior Books.

Jackson, D. (1965-1966). Interoffice memorandum and correspondence pertaining to the creation of the Brief Therapy Center.
• Interoffice memo regarding a proposal being written by Dr. Fisch to estab-

lish a brief therapy clinic and evaluation project, 8-27-1965 (a).
- 2 page interoffice memo to D. Fisch regarding revising the brief therapy research proposal, 11-15-1965 (b).
- A series of interoffice memorandum pertaining to revising the BTC research proposal and potential funding sources, 1-20-1966; 1-27-1966; 2-14-1966.
- Correspondence between Jackson and the Louis B. Hancock Foundation securing $12,000 to fund start up of the Brief Therapy Center, 2-2-1966; 5-4-1966.
- Correspondence between Jackson and Dr. Philip Lee, Asst. Secretary for Health & Human Services, regarding funding of the Brief Therapy Center, 2-11-1966; 2-24-1966.

Lederer, W., & Jackson, D. *Mirages of Marriage*, New York: W. W. Norton.

Loar, L. (1998), Making Tangible Gains in Parent-Child Relationships with Traumatized Refugees, *Intervention*, 2 (3), 210-220.

Nardone, G., & Watzlawick, P. (1993). *The Art of Change*, San Francisco, CA: Jossey-Bass.

Nardone, G. (1995). Brief strategic therapy of phobic disorders: A model of therapy & evaluation research. In J. Weakland & W. Ray (Eds.). *Propagations, Thirty Years of Influence from the Mental Research Institute*, pp. 91-106 New York: Haworth.

Ray, W. (2005) (Ed.). *Don D. Jackson—Essays from the Dawn of an Era, Selected papers volume I*, Phoenix, AZ: Zeig, Tucker, Theisan, Ltd.

Ray, W., & Watzlawick, P. (2005). The Interactional Approach - Enduring Conceptions from the Mental Research Institute. *Journal of Brief Therapy*, 6, (1), 1-20.

Ray, W. & Nardone, G. (Eds.), (2009). *Insight May Cause Blindness and other Essays by Paul Watzlawick*, Phoenix, AZ: Zeig, Tucker, Theisen Ltd.

Schlanger, K., & Anger-Díaz, B. (2005). A new direction for Brief Therapy at MRI—Problem Solving across cultures. *Journal of Systemic Therapies*.

Schlanger, K. & Martin, B. (1998). Who really wants to change? Working briefly with a customer. *The Counselor*, July/Aug., Natonal Ass. Of Alcoholism & Drug Abuse Counselors.

Soo Hoo, T. (2005). Working within the cultural context of Chinese-American Families, *Journal of Family Psychotherapy*, 16 (4).

Watzlawick, P., Beavin-Bavelas, J., & Jackson, D. (1967). *Pragmatics of Human Communication—A Study of Interactional Patterns, Pathologies, & Paradoxes*. New York, W. W. Norton.

Watzlawick, P., Weakland, J., Fisch, R. (1974). *Change—Principals of Problem Formation and Problem Resolution*, NY: WW Norton.

Watzlawick, P. (1976). *How Real is Real?* New York: Vintage Books.

Watzlawick, P. (1978). *The Language of Change*, New York: Basic Books.

Watzlawick, P., & Weakland, J. (Eds.), (1977). *The Interactional View*. New York: W. W. Norton.

Watzlawick, P. (Ed.), (1984). *The Invented Reality*, New York: W. W. Norton.

Watzlawick, P. (1989). *Munchhausen's Pigtail*, New York: W. W. Norton.

Weakland, J. (1970/2007). Introductory comments to lecture by G. Bateson. 1st Don D. Jackson Memorial Conference. Audio recording. Palo Alto, CA: MRI. In Ray, W. (2007). Bateson's cybernetics: The basis of MRI Brief Therapy, *Kibernetics,* 26, (7 & 8), 859-870.

Weakland, J., Fisch, R., Watzlawick, P., & Bodin, A. (1974). Brief therapy: Focused problem resolution. *Family Process*, 13 (1), 141-168.

Weakland, J. (1981). One thing leads to another. *Rigor & Imagination—Essays from the Legacy of Gregory Bateson*, New York Praeger Publishers.

Weakland, J., Ray, W. (Eds.) (1995). *Propagations, Thirty Years of Influence from the Mental Research Institute*, NY: Haworth.

# CHAPTER 1

# Resistance to Change
# in the Psychiatric Community[1]

## *Richard Fisch, M. D.*

As Psychotherapists, we are constantly involved in encouraging change in our patients. In one way or another we devote a major portion of our working lives hoping that we may be of some assistance in the broadening of their experiences in the world. Yet less attention is paid to the broadening out of our own professional lives or the tools we use to help patients achieve changes in themselves. I am sure that most therapists, at some points in their career, have paused to take a backward look over the growth of their work. However, the press of work keeps up and it is difficult to keep questions about one's own development in mind for long. We continue trying to help, using the tools we know best and perhaps not varying them very much until more years go by and again we may pause to look back on our own change, or lack of it.

Some time ago the pressure of working in a clinic overloaded with patients, most of whom lacked sophistication but who were badly in need of help, forced me to reevaluate the techniques I had been trained in, primarily psychoanalytic psychotherapy. I decided to use more symptom-oriented methods which departed widely from my own technical background. It was the reaction of colleagues to these innovations that brought into sharper focus the questions I

---

[1] Originally published in the, *Archives of General Psychiatry*, Vol. 13, 1965, Vol. 13, October, 359-366

raised above: how ready are psychotherapists to change and explore? I decided to condense the experiences with colleagues into some organized form so that other psychiatrists who are starting to settle into their careers might take a backward look a little sooner and to gain some understanding of the difficulty that might be faced in attempting to make alterations in that career.

In order to develop new approaches, psychiatrists at all levels of involvement—training, private practice, hospitals, and research organizations—must be maximally free to entertain, plan, and test new techniques.

In this paper I am concerned with obstacles to the opening up of new pathways; obstacles manifested by orthodoxy, sectarianism, overspecialization, and a shying away from dissension (Thompson, 1958; Rose & Esser, 1960; Hollingshead & Redlich, 1958). The second portion of this paper is devoted to suggestions that can be undertaken at various levels of psychiatric organization in overcoming trends toward stagnation.

## I. Sources

New approaches for dealing with deviant behavior and altering it have run into resistances that stem from multiple sources: the presumption that psychoanalytic concepts are to be the yardstick used to measure new techniques, the evaluation of new ideas by examining the innovator's motivation rather than his ideas, and overt and covert pressures on innovators deriving from the nature of formal and informal psychiatric organizations.

### A. "The Psychoanalytic Yardstick."

When one considers the overall direction of psychiatric training in the United States, there can be little doubt that its principal vector is psychoanalytic, either in its pure form or in some attenuated state (Grinker, 1958).[2] The large mass of private practitioners reflect this trend also. The vocabulary of psychiatry today—unconscious, transference, resistance, orality, anality, etc.—indicates the widespread use of psychoanalytic concepts and methodologies. Other approaches to treatment—somatic therapies, hypnosis (Wolfberg, 1948), behavior therapy, social case work, family therapy, milieu therapy, psychodrama-are usually considered tangents of the main core of treatment, psychoanalytic psychotherapy. Yet no study of results has ever adequately documented the superiority of this method over any of the preceding techniques (Grinker, 1958). Thus the choice of therapeutic method may be unrelated to effectiveness and this has ramifications when clinicians evaluate new techniques. Because of the priority given to psychoanalytic concepts in training and practice, a major source of re-

---

[2] For example, many of the renowned training centers are in some fashion associated with formal psychoanalytic institutes, such as the Menninger Clinic, the Yale Department of Psychiatry, or the New York Psychiatric Institute.

sistance to change in psychiatric approaches is the use of a "psychoanalytic yard-stick" and the following illustrates how it is used.

## B. *"The Dependence on Insight."*

*While* it is not the sale property of psychoanalytic forms of therapy, insight as the sine qua non of behavior change has received its greatest impetus from psychoanalytic theory and practice. The greatest bulk of time spent in treatment revolves more around this one basic assumption than any other approach (such as suggestion, alterations in milieu, directions, etc). Often, insight itself is regarded as the goal of treatment and therapists will report "progress" in patients solely on the acquisition of insight. New methods that do not include insight will therefore be criticized simply on the basis that it does not include this "essential." One experimental therapist, after describing the rapid and apparently durable results achieved in relieving a patient of symptoms through a variant of behavior therapy, was criticized by a more conventional colleague because her symptoms were relieved before she could "get insight into her problems."

## C. *"Transference Culture."*

One phenomenon, stemming from psychoanalytic thought, is that new forms of therapy are often discounted on the basis that results achieved through any wide departure from psychoanalytic therapy are "only transference cures" or "flights into health." Thus, what in all other scientific fields is the essential criterion - results - in psychoanalytic psychiatry is relegated to a secondary position in favor of consistency with a prevailing theory. I have heard therapists claim that, should even symptom relief achieved without insight prove to last the lifetime of the patient, they would still regard it as a transference cure and something less than desirable. The concept of flight into health is also an unfortunate and devastating one. One wonders how often patients who have achieved marked relief and ego enhancement in early stages of treatment are subsequently convinced of the "illusory" nature of their improvement and seduced into lengthy if not interminable treatment with attendant loss of confidence in their ability to gauge improvement because symptom change was labeled as flight into health. Telling patients that we are not interested in results may be a useful stratagem of treatment, but to disregard results in evaluating any form of therapy is dangerous.

Therefore, even if innovators can cite impressive results with new techniques they run the risk of criticism that their methods, in departing from psychoanalytic practice, have achieved results less than desirable, i.e., only transference cures.

D. *"Covert Manipulation by Therapists."*

Psychoanalytically oriented therapists often fail to see their manipulation of patients which is inherent in any interaction, especially in a psychotherapeutic one. Conversations are continually being steered by the therapist not only in obvious ways, such as questions, but often by such subtle clues as variations in attention, manifestations of tension such as changes in breathing, tonal emphases, and even the display of books which indicate the therapist's areas of interest (Rogers, 1960). Thus, while therapists exert covert manipulation of patients, they can continue the myth of "nondirectiveness." Being nondirective or noncommittal has come to be a hallmark of modern psychotherapy, so much so that patients will often state that they realize they should not ask their therapists advice of everyday matters nor expect answers to questions.

As a result of the high value placed on nondirection, and because of the blind spots to covert direction, there is resistance to forms of treatment that involve open directiveness, such as hypnosis, behavior therapy, milieu therapy, etc.

E. *"Questioning Motivation of Clinicians."*

Clinicians would be freer to evaluate the pros and cons of new ideas if they simply focused on the content of those ideas. What does the innovator propose? How does he organize his ideas? How has he applied them? What kind of results has he achieved? These are the questions that should be raised. They are often not raised, and instead there is a preoccupation with what the innovator's motivation was in bringing forth divergent ideas. Again, while not the sole property of the psychoanalytic movement, the impetus for this has come from the priority given to psychoanalytic therapy, especially that of "countertransference." Clinicians who depart from the psychoanalytic yardstick find that colleagues may be more interested in their "countertransference distortions" than in the method and results of any new ideas brought forward. Probably the clearest example of this is found in an editorial letter in the *International Journal of Psychoanalysis* on the very subject of deviance from classic analytic practice:

> If we ask ourselves what may be at the root of such dissidence as presents itself in the phenomenon of the neoanalytic movement, we must come up with answers bearing on the problem of our selection of candidates, and on those qualities of the training analysis and of the supervisory system which eventuate in failure of resolution of *pathological narcissism,* in survival of *narcissistic identification* in the transference and counter-transference, and in the persistence of the *transference neurosis* itself. Our failure to be uncompromising in the application of our psychoanalytic insight into our au-

thoritarian roles as teachers and educators may have something to do with the fact that at least some of our colleagues and students find solace for *narcissistic injury* in alliance as dissident coteries (italics mine). (Gitel, 1962)

Psychoanalysis is burdened with a theory that permits the invalidation of attempts to alter it, as well as disqualify techniques operating outside the analytic framework.

### F. *"Organizational Pressures on Innovators."*

Clinicians who experiment within a formal organization such as a hospital or clinic, are subject to pressures, both open and covert, which may discourage innovation. For example, one of the ward psychiatrists at a local state hospital attempted to reorder his ward using concepts of a "therapeutic community." He was never told to desist, but instead was transferred to one of the chronic services, an oft-used form of censure. In such cases, the resistance to innovation is based not so much on resistance to any particular concept of treatment so much as a perceived threat to the status quo of the hospital.

In more subtle forms, supervisors in residency training programs may discourage innovation by asking that supervisees explore their own motivation for deviation from conventional treatment. Residents who hope to practice in the area in which they are taking their training are particularly vulnerable to this kind of discouragement since they will have to depend on senior clinicians and their hospital for recognition and sources of referral. The same applies to young psychiatrists in the community who also depend on the senior members of the profession to introduce them into the professional community and provide referrals. A reputation for being "far out" may seriously jeopardize the newcomer's practice.

More experienced therapists, at the same time, subject themselves to similar restraints by failing to encourage or allow for discussion of divergent ideas and practices among members of professional societies and hospital staffs. Time that might be devoted to such discussion is frequently taken up with plodding administrative details, or "sociability hours." Often clinical material is relegated to "safe" outside speakers who are freer to present controversial ideas since they are more independent economically and professionally from the hosting group. Since there is probably more innovation by conventional therapists than is apparent, such "off-beat" speakers may encourage innovators simply by demonstrating that respected others are pursuing similar lines. That conventional clinicians depart from "proper" technique is most usually revealed in small "trusted" groups, and as asides, rarely in an open formal meeting. Even so, such asides still allow for the realization that orthodoxy is not all that popular or slavishly followed and younger therapists in particular may soon realize the illusory nature of "standard practice." I am not suggesting that formal professional groups, such as local psychiatric societies, are composed of members all burning for the opportunity to present new and revolutionary ideas, nor, if this were so, that this would be the best use of such societies; but where pertinent issues are strongly felt by many therapists, the airing of these issues is discouraged. For example, in one psychiatric society, several therapists were concerned over the loose and confusing interpretation of psychiatric indications for therapeutic abortion and asked that a panel discussion be held to try to shed some light on the matter. Despite repeated requests, even in the face of programless meetings, no such discussion has been held even though the initial suggestion was raised some two or more years ago.

It also seems difficult for therapists to describe what they do with patients during therapy sessions. At one hospital the psychiatric department was asked to present clinical material at their department meetings much as it is done in other medical and surgical sections. Psychiatrists then rotated in describing their own clinical experiences. However, the descriptions were inclusive of everything except what the therapist himself did. The history of the patient's illness occupied the major bulk of the time; this was followed by the various insights or resistive maneuvers the patient availed himself of, and finally some material related to improvement. Members, both those presenting as well as the audience, seemed uninterested in this form of participation and finally it was done away with altogether. (As a recognition by members of the resistance to revealing one's work, the first presenter was roundly congratulated, not on his presentation, but for the fact that he had the courage to go first and "break the ice.") In no other branch of medicine is there such secrecy as to what the practitioner does with his patient. In hospital practice, the psychiatrist is free from observation of his work which his medical and surgical colleagues accept as a daily part of their routine, and since a consensus of what constitutes successful psychiatric treatment is lacking, even this area is unmonitored.

Finally, there is a tacit acceptance among psychiatrists that while various approaches to treatment are useful, most of these should be left to "specialists" to handle while the average therapist should continue to devote himself to individual psychoanalytic psychotherapy. For example, while most psychiatrists in the local area regard themselves as flexible in approaches to teach patient, this usually means utilizing some variant of psychotherapy with occasional prescribing of psychotropic drugs. For other techniques, patients are referred to the "specialists" in group therapy, family therapy, hypnosis, shock treatment, brief therapy. In this way, therapists avoid testing out, exploring, or understanding newer, divergent methods of treatment and "encapsulate" these to a relatively small number of their colleagues.

## II. Alternatives

In part I, I discussed factors encouraging the resistance to change in psychiatric treatment. These consist of the presumed priority of psychoanalytic methods, the use of psychoanalytic theory as the yardstick by which non-analytic methods are measured, the relegating of results to a secondary position in evaluating techniques in favor of questioning the innovator's motivation, the secrecy surrounding the activity of psychotherapists with their patients, and overt and covert pressures on innovators within formal and informal professional groups. In this section I will suggest alternatives that might be undertaken at various levels of professional experience to combat these stultifying forces.

A. *Alternative: Training Phase.*

1. De-emphasis on Inpatient Experience: The core of training in most residency programs continues to be treatment of hospitalized patients. Further, in the great majority of programs, the psychiatrist-to-be is introduced to the field by working in an inpatient setting and essentially with those people for whom outpatient care and community support has failed. For the three years of formal training, contact with hospitalized people constitutes the great bulk of experience, and the resident has little if any opportunity to appreciate those steps that occurred as the individual was removed from the mainstream of society and thus, he has a poorer chance of evaluating those aspects of mental hospitalization that in themselves retard the individual's return to his role as a community member. The emphasis placed on hospital work gives the resident a lopsided picture of the efforts needed to reduce the cost of mental illness to the individual and his society. It also encourages the fatalism that if the patient does not respond to ordinary treatment methods there is always the hospital. While we ordinarily think of the mental hospital as a retreat for the patient, it also serves as a "retreat" for the psychiatrist, and the newcomer to the field inadvertently learns this in his initial experience. It also places an emphasis on discharge from the hospital as the criterion of therapeutic results rather than on keeping people out of them in the first place. In essence, the emphasis on inpatient experiences fosters an attitude of status-quoism.

*Alternative:* The initial experience in residency training programs should be on outpatient and community facilities and methods used in these settings. Additionally, hospital experience could be relegated to a much smaller percentage of the resident's time, and then, ideally, should involve different types of institutions: state hospitals, private sanitaria, county or local psychiatric wards in general hospitals, day care and night care facilities, and halfway houses. In this way the resident will get some idea of how he may use available inpatient facilities in a controlled and individualistic way.

2. Exposure to Different Treatment Methods: While most programs involve some experience with many types of treatment, the great emphasis seems to be on psychoanalytic forms of psychotherapy. While residents may have some hand in group therapy, milieu therapy, hypnosis, etc., it is primarily in his handling of the psychotherapeutic interview that he will receive supervision and some demand for proficiency. He is led to understand that the most flagrant ineptness in these other procedures will be overlooked if he can demonstrate facility with psychoanalytic/psychodynamic concepts and methods. A priority for these techniques is thus fostered often without regard for the appropriateness to the individual being treated. The other approaches come to be regarded as interesting tricks useful for one to have up his sleeve, but to be used sparingly.

*Alternative:* Residency programs should give greater emphasis to the techniques and rationales of treatment besides the psychoanalytic therapies. Residents should be encouraged to show a proficiency in diverse methods of treatment and should become comfortably familiar with hypnosis, family therapy, group therapy, behavior therapy, brief therapeutic maneuvers, as well as individual psychotherapy.

3. Direct Supervision of Work: The practice in most residency programs is to supervise the resident's work by discussing cases and interviews, relying solely on the resident's own report as to what he is doing. (If the same practice were used, let us say in a surgical residency, there would be chaos.) Yet the psychiatric resident is led to feel that he will not be held too accountable for what he does since little opportunity is taken to view and evaluate his work directly. This helps to foster a "conspiracy of silence" among therapists and to protect each other not only from criticism but also from growth in professional competency. The resident is encouraged to distort reports of his work to fit in with what he perceives to be the expectations of any particular supervisor. There are fewer restraints on his being sloppy with the care and management of patients and his interpersonal dealings with them.

*Alternative:* Direct supervision of what the resident actually does with his patient should become the rule, not the exception: there should be widespread use of observation rooms, sitting with the resident during interviews, tape-recordings, and use of closed-circuit television. As early as possible, residents should get used to such direct observation so that they can develop increasing comfort when their work is closely scrutinized and evaluated.[3]

---

[3] Dr. Alan Sherman contributed this suggestion.

4. Multidisciplinary Supervision: Residents are usually supervised by other psychiatrists. One outcome of this is to confine orientation within a narrow field and to deprive the resident of those approaches developed within the fields of social work, psychology, vocational rehabilitation, and other fields of human study. (Where psychologists' contributions are used, it is most often limited to psychological testing, rarely, if ever, on psychological insights into learning theory, for example.) Contributions by anthropologists and sociologists are hardly ever used. In any event, while some of these personnel may be utilized as adjuncts to treatment, they seldom, if ever, are used to supervise and criticize residents' work. Thus, this limited approach to supervision fosters a narrowness of outlook that residents carry into practice in their later professional lives.

*Alternative:* Residents should be supervised not only by psychiatrists, and preferably psychiatrists of varying clinical orientations, but by other workers in the behavioral sciences: social workers, psychologists, sociologists, anthropologists, and rehabilitation workers.

5. Encouragement of Research and Experimentation: While some residencies encourage research (eg, Stanford University) few incorporate it as a regular requirement for residents. Much lip-service is paid concerning the limitations and incompleteness of psychiatric knowledge as it now stands, but little real attention is given to doing anything about it. Even basic techniques for the setting up of a research problem are unfamiliar to most graduates from a psychiatric residency, and greatly hampers their evaluating of research reported in the literature.

*Alternative:* All residencies should require students to become involved in an appreciable period of research. While it may not be feasible to expect all trainees to come up with original ideas, all trainees can be expected to participate as members of a research team. As much as possible research should be encouraged along "formal" lines utilizing practices of record keeping, controls, statistical validations, etc.

6. Training in Sociology, Anthropology, and Communication Theory: The vast bulk of a resident's formal education is designed to provide acquaintance and mastery of his role as a physician. The growing recognition of social phenomena involved in "mental illness" (Szasz, 1961) requires that psychiatrists have more than a medical and psychopathological orientation to individual and group behavior. Implicit in the work of psychiatrists is an assumption of the individual's conflict with his prevailing social mores and thus, a more disciplined approach is needed in understanding those mores and the varieties of cultural norms, their transmission, and responses by non deviants to infrac-

tions of these norms. In essence, one cannot truly understand the deviations in individuals without an equal study of the group in which he is deviating.

*Alternative:* Some didactic work in sociology, anthropology, and communication theory should be required in all psychiatric residencies. Further, medical schools should encourage the study of at least sociology and anthropology in undergraduate schools by those students planning to enter medicine. Other requirements, such as physics or advanced courses in chemistry could be made optional to allow for time needed for socially oriented studies.

### B. *Alternatives in the Psychiatric Community.*

Earlier I had described factors operating in the psychiatric community that fostered resistances to change. While the resident training experience may be utilized to initiate alternative steps in order that a receptivity towards change can occur, this receptivity must continue when the resident reaches practice and enters his professional community.

1. Restoring an Emphasis on Results: One of the major factors that discourages change is the use of yardsticks for new methods that depend on whether such methods stick to prevailing techniques, rather than on results achieved. Efforts to keep the criterion of results constantly in mind by therapists in the community, therefore, becomes an important focus. The importance of this is discussed in part I, A, B, and C.

*Alternatives:*
(a) One or more meetings of local psychiatric societies should be devoted to discussions of results in therapy. While no hard and fast consensus of opinion can be expected, therapists can nevertheless be encouraged to exchange ideas on their own criteria for results. Merely the placing of such a topic on the agenda would be a step in bringing this aspect of treatment into sharper focus and hopefully force therapists into reexamining their own ideas about it. In particular, the opinions of practitioners of divergent orientations should be solicited. This would give members of the professional community a chance to crosscheck their own ideas with those psychiatrists using hypnosis, group therapies, brief therapies, etc., besides those using psychoanalytically based psychotherapies.
(b) As much as possible, a therapist should be informed by colleagues when his ex-patients have reentered therapy with another therapist. This would provide more data on duration of symptom relief, or the shifting of symptoms. It would be important to know, for example, whether the "markedly improved" patient has sought treatment elsewhere shortly after termination with his original therapist. In our own local setting this practice is rather well adhered to but still retains a sort of informal status

and may be overlooked where the new and old therapists are of appreciably different orientations or are otherwise personally and professionally distant from each other. Also, no effort is made to overcome the resistance of a patient to letting his former therapist know of his reentry into treatment if he has some resentment about his experiences with his former therapist.

(c) The development of follow-up studies should be encouraged as well as their use by all therapists in the area. The practice of assuming all is well after "successful" treatment or the converse after apparent "unsuccessful" treatment is a drawback in assessing the effectiveness of any treatment approach, and without follow-up studies there is no way for a therapist to know the duration of symptom relief, the additional changes in behavior that followed from any symptom relief or alterations in behavior of members of the patient's family. (e.g., whether the wife sought treatment after the patient had an apparently successful outcome of his own treatment). The local psychiatric society can be instrumental in encouraging the development of such studies through discussion as well as in aiding more disciplined efforts by therapists particularly interested in this endeavor.

2. Decrease Mental Hospital Use: Mental hospitalization involves the removal of the individual from his community, not only in a physical sense, but more important in his role as a respected participant, worker, family member, and consumer. Mental hospitalization may also deepen the individual's role as a "patient" and rehabilitative efforts following discharge have to cope with the effects of hospitalization itself, often more so than with any aftermath of the "illness" itself (Goffman, 1961). Things that were taken for granted now become quite important and potentially perilous for the discharge from a mental hospital: application for driver's license, security clearance, job applications, etc. Fits of pique are no longer simple luxuries since they may be interpreted as "he's ready for the hospital again." The ease of reentrance to the hospital is appreciably greater once a person has been admitted his first time. At the same time, the accessibility of hospitals relieves therapists of pressure to provide flexible treatment and maintain the individual in the community. He is enabled to shift responsibility for treatment to the hospital setting while saving face at having failed. "The patient needs hospitalization" is often a rationalization for failure on the part of psychiatric treatment, community resources, and family support.

*Alternative:* Mental hospitals, large and small, should be closed, most feasibly in stages. Whatever supervised living arrangements are needed during crisis situations can be provided by psychiatric facilities in local general hospitals, day-care centers, special residences, and night-care centers. They would enable patients to maintain a much greater physical and social tie with the community and at the same time be geared to short-term stays only to last during a crisis. It would also force therapists to think in terms of "cure," i.e., measures to maintain the individual in the community in as productive and participant roles as possible. Newer approaches to treatment would have more of a chance of being heard and evaluated and with less resistance to adopting them.

Local psychiatric groups as well as lay organizations such as mental health societies, can use their influence and prestige to direct legislation towards these ends. Such influence can also be used to encourage local governmental and private resources to provide for smaller, community based living units such as those described above. In the meantime, there should be awareness that the resorting to mental hospitalization reflects a failure at all levels of community efforts, not an expected phase of treatment.

3. Avoidance of Economic Sanctions: Therapists will be discouraged from developing or discussing innovations if they run the risk of being considered "far out" and thereby suffer their professional standing and, concomitantly, sources of referral. While this need not be a major problem to innovators, since referrals may continue by colleagues in general medicine who may have a more pragmatic approach to patient help, nevertheless, the esteem a therapist is held in by other therapists can make a difference.

*Alternative:* One measure that may reduce the economic impact of deviance is to set up an impartial referral agency. For example, referral sources are often provided by more established and "busier" therapists in the area. "Overflow" that they are unable to treat at anyone time can be shunted to a central referral pool set up by local psychiatric societies, mental health groups, etc. Therapists who have treatment time available could receive referrals on a rotation basis. Needless to say, the patient's consent and privilege to refuse any particular doctor would be honored. Such a plan is in operation in our own local area. Thus, psychiatrists of all persuasions and individuality in approach are enabled to receive referrals without prejudice. This is not a complete answer since therapists are free to bypass such a referral agency, but it does at least reduce economic sanction somewhat.

4. Increase Discussions of Practices by Therapists: As described before, where therapists are reluctant to discuss their own operations as apart from theory they subscribe to, an impression of "conventional" practice is maintained. The aura of "proper technique" is heightened when innovating therapists fail to disclose their innovations and stick to discussions of more ac-

cepted methods. A great deal of highly individualistic and unconventional ideas may remain hidden so that occasional revelations of experimental work may appear more unique than is real. It becomes important for members of the psychiatric community to recognize the degree to which therapists depart from theoretical frameworks in their actual operations with patients. I see no way around this problem other than to encourage members of psychiatric societies and hospital staffs to give clearer pictures of exactly what they do with patients. Admittedly this is no easy road since a concern about being considered "far out" or unorthodox may carry with it professional and economic consequences and therefore invites silence, vagueness, and distortion of one's own operations. It can only be hoped that as the *results* of treatment become more important than the *way* they are achieved, and as innovation becomes more encouraged and sanctions for deviancy become reduced, therapists will feel freer to communicate more fully and accurately.

## Summary

In the foregoing, I have described resistances to new ideas and methods as manifested by psychiatrists individually and in groups, ie, the "psychiatric community." Much of this resistance stems from the priority given to psychoanalytic thought and its use as a yardstick to measure newer techniques. It also stems from a concern about the motivation of innovators rather than a concern about results. The risk of economic and professional sanctions heightens this resistance since it discourages innovators from discussing work with colleagues as well as obscuring the departures from "conventional" theory that many therapists avail themselves of. I have offered alternative suggestions stressing the need for changes in psychiatric training programs but also alternatives applicable to practice and participation in the "psychiatric community."

## References

Gitel, M. (1962). Letter, *Journal of International Psychoanalytic Association*, 43: 375.

Goffman, E. (1961). *Asylums,* Garden City, NY: Anchor Books, Doubleday & Co.

Grinker, R. (1958). "A Philosophical Appraisal of Psychoanalysis," in J. Masserman

(Ed.): *Science and Psychoanalysis*, NY: Grune & Stratton, Inc., Vol 1.

Hollingshead, A., & Redlich, F. (1958). *Social Class and Mental Illness,* NY: John Wiley & Sons.

Rado, S.; Grinker, R.R; & Alexander, F. (1963). Editorial, *Archives General Psychiatry*, 8: 527, June.

Rogers, J.M. (1960). Operant Conditioning in a Quasi-Therapy Setting, *Journal of Abnormal Social Psychology, 60:* 247.

Rose, M., & Esser, M.A. (1960). The Impact of Recent Research Developments on Private Practice, *American Journal of Psychiatry* 117: 429-433 (Nov).

Szasz, T. (1961). *The Myth of Mental Illness,* NY: Paul B. Hoeber, Inc., a division of Harper & Brothers.

Thompson, E. (1958). A Study of the Emotional Climate of Psychoanalytic Institutes, *Psychiatry* 21: 45-52, Feb.

Wolfberg, L.R (1948). *Medical Hypnosis,* NY: Grune & Stratton, Inc., p 12.

# CHAPTER 2

# On Becoming Family Therapists

## Richard Fisch, Paul Watzlawick, John Weakland and Arthur Bodin

In our day everything seems to be pregnant with its contrary.
—*Karl Marx*

Life is a game, of which rule number one is: this is no game;
this is dead serious.
—*Alan Watts*

Like any other professional, the family therapist is threatened by professional deformations, none of which is as insidious as the gradual, almost imperceptible straying from the established doctrine. Very little has as yet been said—let alone published—about these dangers, but we believe that the sounding of a note of warning can no longer be delayed. Our task will not be an easy one, for the phenomena which we have come to identify over the course of many years are subtle and do not readily meet the eye of the critical observer. They are of a multi-faceted nature and can perhaps best be referred to collectively as the Danger of Unbecoming Book Therapists (abbreviated DOUBT), wherein "book" refers to the right theory and technique of family therapy.

By and large, these dangers stem from two different sources, one of which is located in the therapist, the other in his patients. In the give-and-take of the therapy situation, these two influences are bound to be present simultaneously and to overlap, interpenetrate, and compound each other to the point of utter frustration. We present first these two classes of DOUBT phenomena, and then show some of the many ways in which their combination can corrupt the process and outcome of any treatment.

## The Therapist

Talking first about the therapist himself, we find that he is threatened by the ever-present danger of paying more than lip service to the idea that he is not treating individuals, but human relationships and systems formed of such relationships. While no reasonable objection can be raised against a colleague's defending family therapy against the orthodox schools of intrapsychic dynamics by the expedient of frequent references to interaction, systems behavior, and systems pathology, he should nevertheless realize that there is a limit to which he should push this philosophy in his practical work.

Family therapists are an unruly crowd; the quantum jump from their original training to family therapy has proved a heady wine for some of them, who in the seclusion of their private offices are experimenting with ideas of yet another jump, this time from the orthodoxy of family therapy to treatment methods which do not even yet have a name. Revolution as an aim in itself is an ever-present danger—witness the many East Europeans who first fought the Nazis, and then after their liberation fought the Communists. It seems to us that not all of our colleagues possess the moral fiber to resist the temptation of pushing the idea of interaction to extremes, such as taking it quite seriously. Then they are eventually beset by great doubt—or rather, great DOUBT. The main part of this chapter is, therefore, devoted to pointing out where these colleagues are losing contact with the established and accepted theory of family therapy, by what arguments they try to justify their deviations, and how these arguments can best be countered.

## The Patient

The danger which the patients unwittingly bring into the therapy game has been known for some seventy years. Regrettably, we all have become complacent about this danger during the last fifteen years or so. In fact, a recent survey conducted by the New Caledonian Institute of Experimental Psychopathology* shows that references in the literature to this phenomenon have dropped from 86.2% in 1917 to a mere 2.7% in 1968 ($x2 = 17.351$, $p = > .000$)! We are here, of course, referring to the patient's persistent tendency to escape into health, a most exasperating problem, wrecking the successful course of many a well-planned therapy. Over the decades, this phenomenon has lost none of its importance, and it is in this connection that therapists in DOUBT are very likely to display one of their simplistic and yet so subtle sophisms: reduced to its simplest terms, these colleagues argue that if a therapist accepts the patient's complaint as a reason for starting therapy with him, he should by the same logic accept his statement of satisfactory improvement as a reason for terminating treatment. They further argue that there is no evidence in the literature of any crises arising in the lives of patients who stopped therapy simply because they felt better, no matter how their therapist felt. This second argument is especially specious, for one cannot demand the same rigorous evidence for a well-known fact of everyday experience as for a more unusual phenomenon. Indeed, the very absence of documented evidence for the danger of a patient's flight into health proves that this is something known to everybody in the field and hardly requires proof. It is almost as if somebody doubted the universally known fact that red haired people have impulsive personalities, just because this fact has not yet been scientifically researched.

After these introductory remarks and warnings, we are now in a better position to appreciate the complications which arise as soon as the two propensities just described begin to compound each other. We shall next consider a number of particularly crucial issues, but do not claim our presentation to be exhaustive.

## Length of Treatment

An important issue is likely to arise early, usually in the first session— at least one family member will probably ask how long they will all have to come. We, of course, believe in the paramount importance of clear, unambiguous and straightforward communication. Yet, we doubt that you the therapist should come right out and tell them, "Anything from eighteen to thirty-six months." In all likelihood, some family members would create an unpleasant scene by gasping and asking rather pointedly, "Are you kidding?" There are better, less crude ways of firmly implanting in the minds of all concerned your own certainty that family therapy is a long-term, open-ended process of restructuring personalities and changing deep-rooted patterns of communication and of family homeostasis. It is usually best to deal with this question subtly. Announce in a matter-of-fact way, "I have Tuesday at three open now, so that will become our regular hour." One may then inquire about "parental models," the nature of their parents' marriage, how they were raised by their parents, etc. But perhaps the most effective way is to translate all marital or family complaints into forms of "communication difficulty." From long experience we can guarantee that with a minimum of effort you can thereby dispel any naive notions of rapid change—so that even if rapid change were somehow to occur in the course of treatment, the family would themselves realize that they must be doing the right thing for the wrong reason, i.e., that they are merely escaping into health. By no means should the therapist encourage any discussion about concrete goals of treatment, since the family would then know when to stop treatment.

We do not exclude the possibility that circumstances beyond your control may at times force you to embark on a time-limited course of treatment. In these cases, emphasis on professional ethics will assist you to label your service as purely a stop-gap measure, something superficial and of temporary value only, and ease the family into long-term therapy as soon as circumstances will permit.

## Experimenter Bias and All That

The only reason for mentioning these well-known facts is that therapists in DOUBT are very likely to see the length of treatment as at least a partial function of the therapist's conviction that it has to be long. They quote the work of Robert Rosenthal (1966) who showed that the performance of laboratory rats (and of human beings in rat-like situations) depends on the bias (i.e., the basic assumptions and beliefs) of the experimenter. According to his regrettable conclusions, the actual outcome of the experimenter-subject interaction reflects much more the prejudices of the former than the pathology of the latter. Quite independently from Rosenthal, very similar conclusions have recently been reached by Spiegel (1969) .

But this is not all. Certain colleagues of ours are quietly voicing their belief that all theories of psychotherapy have limitations which are logically inherent in their own nature (i.e., the premises of the theory). These colleagues insinuate such limitations are typically attributed to human nature. One of their examples is that in terms of the postulates of psychoanalytic theory, symptom removal without insight must perforce lead to symptom substitution and exacerbation of the patient's condition—not because this is necessarily inherent in the mental makeup of human beings, but simply because the premises of the theory permit no other conclusion. For example, they cite the work of Spiegel (1967), who has claimed to have successfully removed such symptoms without symptom substitution. (No lack of data to the contrary needs to stop us from predicting that untoward effects will show up sooner or later, even if it takes decades.)

Therapists in DOUBT are particularly prone to make such mistakes in their thinking, and this should be a matter for grave concern. We might overlook their tendencies to erroneous methods of practice (nobody is perfect), but they do not even think right; that is serious. The simplicity of their views (which will unfold itself in all its complexity in the following pages) about reasonable goals of treatment, and their unwarranted optimism about the possibilities of change are likely to produce in their patients a typical Rosenthal effect and thus encourage the patients' unhealthy tendency to escape into health before their problems can be explored in depth. No time and space need be wasted to uncover the fallacy of these views. Any well-trained therapist can see it clearly. And most therapists, as well as their patients, have a fairly acceptable view about how deep-rooted the problems they are trying to change are. Yet, there are some who need help and guidance even in this area. A word about problems is therefore called for.

## Difficulties, Problems, and "Problems"

As already mentioned, a patient's wish for change is usually accepted as the reason for taking him into treatment. Beyond this point of agreement, however, we again run into controversy. Engaging in what is strongly suggestive of semantic hair-splitting, some of our colleagues insist on a clear distinction between "difficulties" and "problems." According to them, there are at least three ways in which this distinction can be lost sight of: 1. when the presence of an ordinary difficulty is defined as a problem; 2. when the absence of a difficulty is defined as a problem; and 3. when the presence of a difficulty is denied altogether. Since these views are major challenges to our traditional assumptions of pathology, we want to present the reasoning behind them as objectively as possible, so that the reader can judge for himself as to how absurd they are:

1. There are countless difficulties which are part and parcel of the everyday business of living, for which no known ideal or ultimate solutions exist, and which become "problems" primarily as a result of the belief that there should be an ideal, ultimate solution for them. For instance, some therapists in DOUBT claim the problem is not that there is a generation gap (apparently there has been one for the past five thousand years), but that an increasing number of people have convinced themselves that it should be closed. Similarly, they believe that there is probably no other single book which has caused more havoc to marriages than van de Velde's classic ideal Marriage, compared to which all real marriages are miserable failures.

2. According to these colleagues, an essentially similar situation arises when the absence of a problem comes to be considered a problem. Compared to this, is the opposite side of life's normal mixture of effort and enjoyment,

pleasure and pain, in which someone so firmly holds the view that "life is real, life is earnest," that any occurrence of ease, spontaneity, and pleasure is perceived as signifying the existence of something wrong. The woman who upholds motherhood as a glorious sacrifice, the compulsive husband who lives only for work, are likely to define carefree behavior in others as "irresponsible," and therefore a "problem." In such cases, "no sweat" becomes something to sweat about even more.

3. Finally, they say that "problems" can arise out of the denial of undeniable difficulties. While alternative 1. acknowledges the existence of a difficulty, but insists that there must be a perfect solution, here we are faced with a basic contention: there is no difficulty and anybody who sees one must be bad or mad. This allegedly is done by people who refuse to see the complexity of our own highly complex and inter-dependent modern world and define this blindness as a "real," "genuine," and "honest" attitude toward life—thereby labeling those who struggle with these difficulties as uptight hypocrites or exploiters.

The specific ways in which therapists in DOUBT imagine these very ordinary and common views to lead to particular acute or even chronic "problems" will be described a little later, in connection with the goals of their treatment.

A moment's consideration will show where this kind of thinking would take us. First of all, what is the patient to think of a therapist who refuses to see a problem as a problem and calls it a difficulty for which no known solutions exist? He will either be encouraged to escape into health or else is likely to start looking for another therapist. Nothing needs to be said about alternative 2. We are all only too familiar with the effects of such insidious redefinitions of established moral values. Only as far as alternative 3. goes, it does not have much of a chance to cause harm in an era in which encounter groups, politicians, and the military breed such a profusion of two-dimensional thinkers (or, as the French have come to call them since May and June of 1968, *terribles simplificateurs*).

## What? Instead of Why?

It is not difficult to see that this approach to problems is anti-historic and simply overlooks the paramount importance of causation. Here again we run into a subtle sophism: these colleagues do not question the fact that any behavior in the present is shaped and determined by experiences in the past. But they flatly deny that for the purposes of therapy there is essential value in discovering the relation between causative events in the past (pathogenesis) and the present condition (pathology), let alone in the need for the patient himself to grasp this connection, that is, to attain insight. They are even likely to disbelieve that any elucidation of the past has ever made the slightest difference to a patient's present condition. They are sarcastic about what they call the self-sealing argument that the absence of improvement in the present "proves" that the past has not yet been sufficiently explored and understood. To use their own reasoning: they are interested in the ways people are behaving in the here and now, instead of why people behave the way they behave. Basing their work, as they do, to an excessive degree on systems theory, they claim to have found clinical confirmation of von Bertalanffy's concept (1962) of equifinality, purporting that a system's behavior can be quite independent of its initial conditions and determined only by its present parameters. For them the current state of a system is its own best explanation, and they thus show a shocking disregard for insight as the conditio sine qua non of therapeutic change. One of their favorite comparisons is that of a man who, not knowing the game of chess, travels to a country whose language he does not understand and comes upon two people engaged in an obviously symbolic activity—they are moving figures on a board. Although he cannot ask them for the rules and the purpose of the game, a sufficiently long period of watching their behavior will enable him to deduce the lawfulness underlying their interaction. This, they stress, he manages to do without any knowledge of the past or of the inner states of the players, or of the "meaning" of their game. Of course, if he wanted, he could have fantasies about that meaning, but they would have the same significance for his understanding of this two-person system as astrology has for astronomy.

Having thus cavalierly dispensed with insight as the precondition for change, the question arises: how do therapists in DOUBT try to bring about change? The answer, blunt, simple and shocking, is: by something they call direct intervention, but we must plainly label "downright manipulation."

## To Thine Own Self Be True

It is generally accepted that a therapist's attitude must be one of complete honesty, that he should always say what he believes (and even believe what he says), that his communications should be open, clear, straightforward, and guileless, and that he should share his own feelings, problems, and anxieties with his patients. This is particularly true of family therapists, and it is refreshing to notice the growing trend toward using the sessions for an exploration of their own hang-ups, and of experimenting with additional techniques of honesty and spontaneity, such as nude sessions (barring, of course, any expression of sexuality). The effect on their patients must be immeasurable.

In stark contrast to all that, certain colleagues of ours seem almost proud to play chameleons; they employ something akin to judo techniques, using the nature and direction of a human system's pathology to bring about its own downfall. Thus, instead of disarming their patients with the counterthrust of their sincerity, they are likely to yield and in yielding, to manipulate. Like their hypothetical chess observer, they study the rules of a human system's game, asking themselves: "What are these people doing to each other?" not "Why are they doing it?," and then do not shy away from even the most questionable direct interventions into the system's behavior. These colleagues are thus not true to their own selves, although it cannot perhaps be denied that in an odd way they are true to the patients' selves—very much like a good hypnotist who utilizes whatever the subject himself brings into the session by way of expectations, superstitions, fears, and resistances, rather than monotonously applying the one method which is most congenial to himself.

There exists, indeed, a large bag of tricks from which manipulative therapists can draw. They can meet the need of patients who believe in the magical by offering a magical rationale for improvement; they can oblige those who come into therapy in order to defeat the expert, by insisting that real improvement is impossible; they may heap responsibility on the incarnate caretaker until he demands to be taken care of himself for a change; they provide subtle challenge to those who challenge openly; they outdo the confirmed pessimist by sadly commenting on the unrealistic optimism of his views; and to the woman endangered by her own longstanding game of suicidal threats against her family, they may even offer helpful suggestions for a pretty funeral. It must be noted that despite their apparent "flexibility," in all these manipulations, in their frequent use of multiple therapists and assignments of so-called "homework" to patients, these therapists in DOUBT keep harping on a theme of influencing behavior by employing paradox, instead of being rigidly honest and straightforward whatever the costs. Nowhere does this slippery attitude become more manifest than in their outlook on the goals of therapy.

## Goals

While different schools of therapy set themselves different goals, a few common traits can be discerned. Most of us would agree that the outcome of treatment should be in the direction of what has variously been termed genital organization, individuation, heightened sensitivity, self-actualization, improved communication, or merely a positive attitude toward life. In this area we need not fear disagreement from our patients, even though in their lay language they may use more primitive terms. Thus, when asked what they expect from therapy, they may explain that they do not get enough out of life, that they would like to be happier, or especially that in their family they do not communicate. Although expressed in an unsophisticated way, these definitions are useful: they are broad enough to be all-inclusive, they permit an open-ended course of treatment and therefore leave room for spontaneous change, and they take into account the complexity of human beings, with their reasons behind reasons behind reasons. Are we not all familiar with the patient who only wants to stop biting his nails, but is unwilling to consider his deep-seated oral aggressive impulses? Or the parents who complain about the misbehavior of a child, but are blind to the subtle breakdowns of their communication and have difficulty learning how to communicate clearly and openly about all subjects, including their own sexual fantasies? We are familiar with all this— but not those in DOUBT.

They contend that when therapists regard problems as complex, firmly entrenched, reflecting limited patient or family resources, and requiring extensive or intensive change, treatment is likely to be complex, profound, severely restricted by limited patient resources, long in duration, and uncertain in outcome. Using the Rosenthal effect positively, they contend that change can be effected most easily and rapidly if the goal of treatment is reasonably small and refers to a clearly stated and well delimited area of a human system's behavior. They have to admit that this approach seems insensitive to the big, deep, and basic problems which some patients want to talk about, but which are so broad and vague that they perpetuate themselves by this very fact. Indeed, so our colleagues speculate, more often than not a patient's problem lies in the fact that he says he has a problem.

The setting of reasonable, reachable goals—stated as concretely and specifically as possible—thus becomes one of their most important steps, to be taken at the very beginning of treatment. Our colleagues claim that in this task many of Alfred Adler's postulates about life styles and goals (Adler, 1928, 1956) are of immediate relevance to their approach. They also believe they have shown that these goals can be reached in ten sessions or less with a wide variety of patients, and that once a patient has experienced a small change in the seemingly monolithic structure of his "real" problem, this experience of change then generates further, self-induced changes in other areas of his life.

Obviously, very little needs to be said to counter these assumptions and claims. As pointed out in earlier sections, they are anti-historic and anti-causal, but now we see that they also disregard a patient's manifestations of his intrapsychic and unconscious dynamics, as well as the deepest levels of family pathology.

Having disregarded these cornerstones of psychotherapeutic theory, our colleagues feel free to view even the longstanding nature of symptoms, not as chronicity in the usual sense of a basic structural defect in an individual or a family, but as the result of poor handling of everyday difficulties. Again, we shall let their simplistic views speak for themselves:

"Everyday difficulties" are considered those arising most commonly during the normal transitional stages in the careers of individuals and families, when shifts in family functioning and re-definitions of relationships become necessary. These transitions occur most often at certain specific points in time, e.g., from courtship to marriage, from the partial commitment to marriage to a fuller commitment at the arrival of the first child, from autonomy over the children to the surrender of part of that autonomy on the child's entrance into school, and even more so as the child becomes involved with peers in the adolescent period, from a child oriented marital relationship back to a two-party system when the children leave home, from the work-scheduled marital arrangement itself to retirement or to widowhood and its single life (or from marriage to divorce), etc. At any one of these junctures a mishandling of the necessary adjustments is possible, and likely to perpetuate and exacerbate itself.

## The Game Without End

They argue that the way people perpetuate their problems by trying to resolve them in inappropriate, if time-honored, ways is the most important single vicious cycle that they have been able to observe in their work. This pattern can perhaps best be described as the presence of positive instead of negative feed-back loops. For instance, the typical rebellious teenager, when faced with parental discipline, will increase his rebelliousness, which in turn is likely to increase repressive action by his parents, which in turn makes the teenager more rebellious, etc. A similar pattern is often at work between a depressed patient and his family – the more they try to cheer him and make him see the positive sides of life, the more the patient is likely to get depressed. In all of these cases the action which is meant to alleviate the behavior of the other party in actual fact aggravates it, but this fact usually remains outside the awareness of everybody involved, and thus the "remedies" they apply are likely to be worse than the "disease." They behave very much like two sailors hanging out from either side of a sailboat in order to keep it from heeling over. The more one sailor leans overboard, the more the other will be forced to lean out himself, while the boat actually would be quite steady if it were not for their acrobatic efforts at "steadying it."

In this anti-historic, anti-causal view, then, problems are seen as always existing in the here and now, to have their own lawfulness and to perpetuate themselves by their own momentum, so to speak. Poor handling of any everyday problem will tend to lead to more of the same, and this process will inexorably place ever-narrowing constraints on, and produce increasing blindness for, the alternative solutions which are potentially available at all times. People in such a situation are caught in a Game Without End (Watzlawick, 1967), a system governed by increasingly rigid rules but without rules for the change of its rules. Indeed, the inability of human systems to generate from within themselves these meta-rules is, for our colleagues at least, the only useful criterion of pathology. This brings us back to the kind of therapy they practice and advocate.

## Therapeutic Interventions

If pressed for an answer as to how they expect to bring about change, having discarded most principles of psychotherapy and, in particular, of family therapy, therapists in DOUBT are likely to claim that a Game Without End can be broken up only by the introduction of new rules into the system. They are, therefore, particularly interested in studying how systems occasionally reorganize themselves as the result of an almost fortuitous outside event. For example:

On her first day of nursery school attendance a girl of four threw such a tantrum as her mother was preparing to leave that the mother was forced to stay with her for the whole school session. The same happened on the next and all following days, and the situation turned into a severe strain on the mother's (and the teacher's) emotions and time. After about two months and before the school psychologist had a chance to take care of the case, the mother was one morning prevented from taking the child to school. The father drove her over, left her, and went on to work. The girl cried a little, but quickly calmed down and never made a scene again, although the mother resumed taking her to school the following morning. Of course, it could be argued that this was not a case of "real" pathology, but be this as it may, there can be little doubt that the case would have taken a very different course had it been given the label of "school phobia" and treated routinely, exploring the symbiotic relation between mother and child, the marital problem of the parents, and the family's modes of communication, etc.—perhaps even a chance to discover "minimal brain dysfunction" was missed.

Another example of a spontaneous remission that our colleagues claim proves their assumption that a system is its own best explanation and that change can occur quite independently from the historic evolution and the deeper meaning of a symptom is the following:

An unmarried, middle-aged man, suffering from an agoraphobia, had reached the point where his anxiety-free territory had become so small that even the most routine aspects of his daily life could no longer be carried out. He eventually decided to commit suicide by driving to a mountain top, about fifty miles from his home, convinced that after a drive of just a few blocks a heart attack would put him out of his misery. To his amazement and utter elation, he not only arrived safely at his destination, but for the first time in many years found himself completely free from anxiety and has remained so for the last five years.

What our colleagues regard as most noteworthy about this example is the strong paradoxical element of this spontaneous remission which reminds one of the Zen tenet according to which enlightenment comes only after the seeker has given up any hope of reaching it.

At this point, we hope the reader will be sufficiently warned as to the nature and insidiousness of DOUBT. The contagion of DOUBTer's can best be controlled by early recognition and prevention of its spread. Toward that end, we will now describe in more concrete detail the handling of two cases by therapists woefully infected with DOUBT. Read, and let the reader beware! The grim and appalling evidence speaks for itself:

The mother of a fifteen-year-old boy called to seek help. She mentioned on the phone that the boy was overly defiant and hostile to her, but even more so to her husband and, in general, difficult to control, not helping with chores around the house, etc. She implied that her husband's passivity and obtuseness contributed greatly to the alienation between him and the boy. Despite the fact that the therapist could easily recognize the situation as basically a marital one, he naively asked the mother to come in alone! In the initial session she described the problem with the son in greater detail, but included a great deal of not very veiled dissatisfaction with the husband: his lack of leadership in the home, his limited efforts at increasing the family income, and his aloofness toward her. She could sympathize with the boy for his anger and alienation, yet she herself was frustrated by the boy in her attempts to gain his cooperation at home. Book therapists will immediately recognize that the marital conflict was most important; that obviously the son was playing out the mother's hostility toward her husband and that the husband's passivity with the child served as a retaliation against his wife. The husband should have been called in and this central pathology explored. But what did our "DOUBTer" do? He gave priority to the mother's frustration with the son. To test out her readiness to deal more harshly with the son, he told her a joke—that "mental illness is inherited; you can get it from your children." She laughed quite openly at this and began to reveal punitive fantasies she had toward the son She explained that she had felt quite angry, but had dealt with him too leniently for fear of alienating him and thereby losing all parental control.

What follows is hard to believe. The therapist suggested that she depart from honest, straightforward, direct discipline and use subterfuge, double deal-ing, and sabotage! Specifically, she was instructed to complain to her son about her husband (in the second session the husband, in the wife's presence, was instructed to criticize any advice or recommendation that the mother made to the son). She was also asked not to cajole or threaten her son; all wishes for correct behavior were to be made as quiet, simple requests, with the reminder that, "I can't make you do that, but I wish it." If the son did not comply, the mother was then to use unobtrusive sabotage—to put lots of salt in his choco-late pudding, or sand in his bed, or "misplace" a treasured possession of his, etc. If any complaint were raised by the son, she was instructed to play dumb and helpless and apologize profusely for her "absent-mindedness."

In the second session, the one also attended by the husband, he was filled in as to the wife's instructions and he was asked to help her by devising other means of sabotage since his experience as a boy and man could add useful hints to the mother's implementation of this program. In front of the husband she was re-instructed to make the relationship between son and father quite difficult by complaining about her husband, and the husband was told that this was necessary since any ultimate improvement of the father-son relationship could be meaningful only if it were not made easy, especially not by the mother, and that her attempts to keep father and son apart would actually con-stitute a help in the long run.

We think the reader can see enough of the duplicity, insensitivity, and gim-mick employed in this case. It is inconsequential that the son became more tractable at home, that the husband became more openly assertive with his wife, and that she was making efforts to supplement the family income through part-time work. Results are not the most important thing, and should always be treated as secondary to understanding, deeper experiences, height-ened sensitivity, and awareness.

Now, should the reader have assumed that such DOUBTing is limited to marital and child behavior problems, consider the following case:

A woman in her fifties came in for help because her twenty-five-year old chronic schizophrenic son seemed on the verge of another psychotic break. Since the age of fifteen, when he had been diagnosed as schizophrenic, he had spent the majority of his time in mental hospitals and had been in almost con-tinuous treatment with a succession of psychotherapists. The son was asked to come in with her on the second visit, and he displayed the mannerisms and speech characteristics of schizophrenia. The therapist was naive and callous enough to tell him to stop talking "crazy" if he wanted to be understood – and the unfortunate patient complied. He then described some power struggles he got into with his parents, especially his mother. These struggles usually cen-tered on how much money he was to receive and when. Essentially he felt that he was entitled to more allowance and on a much more definite basis. The mother felt that his questionable mental state made it unfeasible to just hand over money which he might squander, and she felt it more appropriate to dole out money on a week-by-week basis, never indicating in advance how much it might be. It appeared to the therapist that her major criterion for doling out money was the son's psychotic behavior, but her reluctance to come across inclined the son to utilize even more psychotic behavior. The therapist then instructed the son to deliberately utilize his psychotic behavior, explaining that since the son felt helpless to contend with his parents' intransigent refusals to comply with his monetary wishes, he had every right to defend himself by threatening to cause an even greater expenditure on their part by his having to go to a mental hospital again. The therapist suggested that this threat could best be conveyed by turning on the psychotic behavior. He made a few comments on what this behavior should look and sound like, comments which were mostly along the lines of what the patient was doing anyway.

This kind of case and its handling is most disturbing: there was no regard for the sensitivity of the schizophrenic son, no attempt made to translate the richness of his metaphoric speech, no exploration of the mother's dependency -overprotectiveness. There was little attempt to get the father in (one telephone call had been placed to him and he refused to come in to see yet another of the son's many therapists, saying that he had "had it"). No explorations were made into any of the many, many possible areas of the family dynamics. These were all ignored by the DOUBT therapist, who proceeded to make only the most crass and superficial interventions. Again, the fact that the mother no longer felt intimidated by the son's psychotic behavior, that she decided to avoid the constant struggle over money and simply arrange that a larger amount be paid on a definite basis, or the fact that the son saved this money until he purchased a car, which in turn gave him greater independence from the mother who had acted as his constant chauffeur—none of this is significant in the face of the therapist's depriving the family of the rich and rewarding experience of exploring, investigating, discussing, and understanding the depths of their family dynamics and its probable rottenness, which should, of course, have received the highest priority, regardless of the time and anguish that this would have entailed.

## Final Warnings

Whenever the reader who wishes to remain a book therapist is approached by a therapist who talks about specific goals of therapy, of strategies and tactics of therapy, of frank manipulation, of shortening therapy time, of dealing with family problems by seeing only one member of the family, and who concerns himself with concrete results, that reader should be most on guard. He is very probably dealing with a DOUBT therapist. Yet some of them can be quite convincing, influential, and even worse. Some therapists in DOUBT get so carried away with their fantasies that they begin to view problems of behavior in the wider social world—in schools, business organizations, social agencies, even politics and government—in a similar simplistic fashion. One shudders to think where this might lead. It is therefore especially important to scotch this trend before its infection spreads. To this end, we offer a few helpful methods for discrediting and dismissing the DOUBTers' arguments and statements, to save oneself and the public from total contamination:

1. Remind yourself and him that what he is saying is not really new or different—that it is something rather traditional, only phrased in new words. Cite supporting and authoritative references.

2. Tell him that you have already tried what he has been talking about and that while it was of mild interest, it was not really effective and you discarded it long ago.

3. Tell him that while what he says is intriguing, it really requires a charismatic (or some other deviant, perhaps psychopathic) character to do it effectively, or to want to do it at all, and that this obviously excludes you since you are normal.

4. After he has gotten through fully explaining the rationale for his innovations, insist that he is leaving out the one fundamental basis for his assumption and imply that if he were to state it, it would simply be a book assumption already in use.

5. As a last resort, nod approvingly throughout his explanation and finish it by ignoring the chronic cases and saying quite cheerfully that indeed you have long been convinced of the important place that "crisis intervention" plays in the armamentarium of treatment as a stop-gap until real therapy can tackle the basic, underlying problems.

Good luck!

# References

Adler, A. (1928), *Uber den nervosen Character*, 4th ed. Munich: Bergmann.

Adler, A. (1956), *The individual Psychology of Alfred Adler*. New York: Basic Books.

Rosenthal, R. (1966), *Experimenter Effects in Behavioral Research*. New York: Appleton-Century-Crofts.

Spiegel, H. (1967), Is symptom removal dangerous? *American Journal of Psychiatry*, 123: 1279-1283.

Spiegel, H. (1969), The "ripple effect" following adjunct hypnosis in analytical psychotherapy. *American Journal of Psychiatry*, 126:91-96.

von Bertalanffy, L. (1962), General systems theory: a critical review. *General Systems Yearbook*, 7:1-20.

Watzlawick, P., Beavin Bavelas, J., and Jackson, D. (1967), *Pragmatics of Human Communication*. New York: Norton.

# CHAPTER 3

# "The Double-Bind Theory" By Reflexive Hindsight[1]

## John H. Weakland

Since the double-bind theory was first propounded—or, sticking more to simple description, since the original publication by Bateson, Jackson, Haley and me of "Toward a Theory of Schizophrenia" (Bateson, Jackson, Haley, & Weakland, 1956)—there has been, if not a scientific earthquake, at least a fair amount of commotion largely traceable to this work.

For example: There is this present book, itself only the latest and most considerable of a series of publications relating to the original article. (Many, though not all, of these writings are listed in Olsen's (1972) review.) Such published works are the most substantial evidence of the paper's impact, or at least the sort of evidence taken most seriously according to scientific and professional conventions of significance. There is also, however, continuing oral discussion of the double bind in the family and Psychiatric fields and various utilizations of the idea in treatment of patients. There is even some noticeable entrance of the term "double bind" into everyday language. Such an impact appears rather striking, especially in a time when there is so much scientific research and publication, in addition to an enamours amount of published writings of more general interest. Amid this mass of words, few new ideas create any lasting stir—though many, for related reasons of widespread commu-

[1] Originally published in *Family Process*, 18 (3), September, 269-277.

nication, blaze up and burn out quickly or are preserved only within some devoted but limited cult.

Moreover, this impact has not been simple and straightforward, but complex and confusing. Some of the publications provoked by the original article support or extend it, but many oppose it—ranging from those that purport to disprove "the double-bind theory" to those that reinterpret its relevance rather sweepingly.

All this is especially interesting to me, as one of the original double-bind authors, and the more so because I note a related curiosity in my own professional life. For ten years I have written nothing further on the double bind, or even anything labeled as directly related to it. I have not even talked about it appreciably, except in discussions of a rather historical slant, usually, with students; e.g.. "How the double-bind concept arose and developed in the context of the Bateson group's research." Yet I see much of my ongoing work—in several rather different areas—as importantly related to the double-bind idea, even if not explicitly referring to it, and I have remained quite interested in what others were writing about the double bind, with recurring thoughts of adding my own latter day two cents' worth. It seems the time for this has finally come.

My aim here, then, is to sketch my own reconsideration of "Toward a Theory of Schizophrenia" and, hopefully, to clarify this murky situation somewhat. The "hindsight" of my title refers, obviously, to this reconsideration. "Self-reflexive" is less obvious; it refers to the fact that the viewpoint from which I will be considering "Toward a Theory" largely derives from the article itself—or at least is consonant with some main principles therein, which over time have become progressively more pervasive and important in my own thinking and acting. Therefore, describing my present view of "Toward a Theory" will, I hope, concurrently make plain my viewpoint for observation, without going over similar ground twice. Such an approach may appear to some as tautological and subjective. My own position on this, however, is very different. It is based on the belief that views—conceptualizations, in fancier language—are all we really have to work with in ordering life experience, even in that part of it called science. If so, the best we can do is to make those views that are used clear and explicit. This has not always been the case in writings on the double bind. Instead, "the double-bind theory" has often been examined and discussed within some context of broad assumptions and premises, including conventions of scientific outlook and beliefs about "theories" and "facts" that were simply taken for granted, or at most implicit. While it may be impossible ultimately to define one's viewpoint and assumptions completely explicitly— and in many situations there may be no great need to attempt this steps toward this ideal goal can be especially useful in instances, like the present one, that are marked by confusion and contradictions.

This account will, by necessity, overlap some prior writings on the double bind, since existing discussion of this subject is already extensive and varied. Yet this account will also, by a combination of necessity and choice, be partial. Not every aspect of "Toward a Theory of Schizophrenia" will be considered here. In the first place, that article involved many ideas and observations, varying both in particular focus and in level of abstractness and generality. Some of these were more fully developed than others; in addition, what was most explicitly stressed in the article and what has proven most significant—in my view—are not necessarily identical. Second, as the joint work of four authors who, despite shared interests and close working relationships, were four quite different individuals, this article does not really present one fully integrated point of view. Rather, it involves a common core plus diverse fringes of emphasis and direction and perhaps even some fringes of disagreement. In these circumstances, I believe it is more useful to concentrate on what I see as the most important features of the original work than to attempt to trace and consider all of its various threads. For related reasons this account will, by choice, be brief, in an attempt to make the main features of "Toward a Theory"— according to this admittedly partial view—stand out with maximum clarity, unobscured by secondary detail.

So much for framing and disclaiming; now for the matter itself. My point of departure is the question. "What is 'Toward a Theory of Schizophrenia' about?" This may seem a silly question. The answer appears obvious: the title, the main content, and much of the subsequent discussion of this article combine to indicate that it is about schizophrenia, something called the double bind, and a theory relating the two. Nevertheless, I think this obvious answer is too simple, narrow and specific. Schizophrenia was indeed the concrete object of inquiry, but here, as elsewhere, a labeled "entity" may be considered in itself, in terms of its more general relevance, or both. And I consider that, while schizophrenia was the specific subject matter, most fundamentally and generally our article was concerned with relationships between behavior and communication, and especially with an approach to investigating these areas of interest.

It is understandable that considerable confusion and misunderstanding might exist on this point. Certainly the article itself made the specific focus explicit and failed to state the more general one as plainly; perhaps it was not even plain in our minds. In addition, the fact that schizophrenia was the particular subject of our work may itself have promoted an overly narrow view of "Toward a Theory." Schizophrenia then was, and largely still is, seen as a great and pressing practical problem. And pressing problems—whether schizophrenia, cancer, or war—tend to be focused on as such, narrowly. An answer to the particular problem is sought, not its implications elsewhere and more broadly.

Yet in other important respects, the focus on schizophrenia was both appropriate and fortunate. Whatever schizophrenia may be—and even if it is not a specific thing at all—it plainly involved behavior that is varied, extraordinary, and "irrational." Such a subject is difficult to investigate and clarify, but any understanding gained is likely to have correspondingly sweeping scope; study of the "abnormal" has repeatedly proved illuminating for the "normal" as well.

"Toward a Theory," in the first place, treated schizophrenia as behavior, both conceptually and empirically. Today this sounds rather simple, perhaps even obvious, at least among those with an interactional orientation. But this view is not accepted everywhere even now, and it certainly was not common then. At that time, by being labeled as definitely a "pathology"' and "irrational," schizophrenia was essentially set off and separated from behavior in general and was defined negatively—in terms of how it was not "normal." In consequence, rather little attention was paid to observing and defining schizophrenia in terms of its own positive characteristics. What it was like was taken as almost obvious, and attempts to explain its existence and nature commonly moved quickly, and largely by inference, into non-behavioral realms whether these were mentalistic or physiologic. In contrast, to consider schizophrenia seriously—even if tentatively—as behavior made for many significant differences in its study and understanding.

The first step then became the more careful recording and examination of schizophrenic behavior as such—actions and especially speech—with the aim of characterizing this behavior more clearly and systematically in positive terms, and terms relatable to more familiar behavior or behavior generally. Such a concern also implied that one should focus attention on not what is most striking and dramatic, nor what is pre-supposed necessarily important, but what is observably basic—that is, regular and general features and interrelationships. This shift of approach was exemplified in the article discussion of how much schizophrenic speech resembles ordinary metaphor except that it is not labeled as metaphor in conventional ways.

This line of inquiry and explanation also implied that "normal behavior" itself may also require fresh observation and better characterization than, for instance, simple ideas of "rationality" provide. Indeed, the consideration of metaphor already began this move and was pursued further, though not altogether explicitly elsewhere in "Toward a Theory"—for example, in discussion of humor, poetry, fiction, and hypnosis.

Beyond the question of "What sort of behavior is schizophrenia?" though closely related to it, lies the question of explaining its nature and occurrence: "How does this sort of behavior come about?" Here, rather than hastening to infer the underlying basis of "schizophrenic thought" from a few scraps of patients' speech isolated from their circumstances, a behavioral view led us to at least examine the occurrence of schizophrenia as one might other behavior—that is, by study of its behavioral contexts. The efforts of "Toward a Theory" in this direction were somewhat divided between consideration of possible learning contexts in the schizophrenic's developmental history and examination of the immediate interactional context of communication. While these two lines of inquiry and explanation are fundamentally similar in their focus on attempting to relate behavior to actual communication that is at least potentially observable, this dual emphasis in the original article certainly has been one source of confusion and uncertainty. The relative importance of the two was never settled—or even clearly postulated—in "Toward a Theory," and in fact this remains a matter of dispute both among the authors and more widely. Perhaps the most that can be said even now is to suggest that, before turning toward what is less directly observable, thorough study of the importance of the present, directly observable context, is most in line with the principles of behavioral study generally.

To study the relationship of behavior and communication, however means that not only the behavior but the communication involved must be handled adequately—again both conceptually and empirically. Indeed, in my estimation "Toward a Theory" made headway in understanding schizophrenia largely because it developed and utilized a new general view of communication. This view involved a number of different but closely interrelated elements. First, there was the beginning of a close identification of communication and behavior as two sides of one coin, so to speak—recognition that the most important aspect of social behavior is its communicative effect and that communication is the major factor in the ordering of behavior socially. In pursuing these connections, "Toward a Theory" certainly took a one-sided or unidirectional view at important points—for example, in seeing a "binder" as imposing a double bind on a "victim." Nevertheless, even if less clearly and explicitly, the article also promoted a view of communication as pervasively and basically interactional—as a system, in which unidirectional *attributions* and various punctuations occur but in which these (even our own) should be seen only as aspects of the larger system. Again, as with schizophrenic behavior itself, what is important for understanding is to see the general pattern of communication, not specific events or messages however dramatic or striking, in isolation. In fact, this whole approach proposed that there is no such isolated event or message. Not only should messages by various parties be seen in relation to one another, there is also no simple message even by one party. "Toward a Theory" pointed out that every message involves multiple channels of communication, modifying one another. Their relationships form a vital part of the pattern, whether they are congruent or contradictory, they must be taken into account jointly. This complexity of messages was considered and examined in various ways in terms of framing, qualification and disqualification, the Theory of Logical Types, stylized types of communication, and others. Perhaps there are better ways yet to be conceived: the important point made was that *somehow* this complexity must be recognized and grappled with as a major feature of communication in itself, that it can only be misleading to fix on one aspect of a communication or a series of aspects separately—as the real or important matter and scant the rest or their interaction. Within this general framework, what is significant in particular, and how, can only be found out by empirical study. Like the pattern called a double bind, what is significant may not be—probably will not be, or it would have been noted before—evident in advance. Rather, it is likely to be subtle and unnoticed, or visible but apparently trivial.

Finally, our viewpoint emphasized the influential aspect of communication as most important and inclusive. The germ of this already existed in Bateson's idea that every message is both a report and a command. That is, there is more than "information," in the common but limited sense of "facts," on the basis of which the receiver may decide action—a view related to the old rationalistic conception of behavior. Communication, with its multiplicity of messages, involves other forms of influence as well, and the whole must be examined. How? Essentially, again, by the only way that is possible to go from the general orientation to specifics—by empirical study focused on effects. What behavior appears to follow a given sort of communication, or, more precisely, what patterns of association of communication and behavior are actually observable? "Toward a Theory" certainly did not settle this question for communication and behavior generally, perhaps not even for schizophrenia and double binds. But it *raised* the question in such a way that it could usefully be pursued, and took some first steps.

This lead, in conclusion, to what I see as central in evaluating "Toward a Theory." This article is a statement of certain observations and ideas, mainly about communication. It is, therefore, a communication about communication. It could, of course, still be judged from some external viewpoint—hopefully, one made explicit—but I have chosen to consider this particular communication here in terms of its own general view of communication. In these terms, this article, like any other communication, involved both reports—observations—and commands—proposals for a viewpoint. To judge it on the basis of its reports alone—inquiry as to "the truth of the theory" being a specific instance of this—is to take a limited standpoint and one which is at odds with the main thrust of the article itself. Man does not live by truth alone, but by ideas and influences. Man does not treat problems by truth alone. An interpretation of behavior—"His criticism is an expression of his loving concern for you"—may be helpful in easing a difficult situation, even if its truth can never be determined. Man does not even pursue science by truth alone. The best hypotheses are "true"—that is, survive tests aimed at disconfirmation—only within certain limits, and this limited truth ordinarily is achieved only late in the development and the consensual *definition,* of a field. "Toward a Theory" is more an opening wedge, proposing a new way of conceptualizing and observing old problems (cf. Kuhn, 3). Although I believe that the observations reported in "Toward a Theory" are reasonably reliable, in such a situation especially (though not exclusively) the accuracy of specific statements may easily be less important than the general direction and viewpoint delineated— just as the general concern of the article with behavior and communication may be more important than its specific concern with schizophrenia. This, perhaps, is not far from Bateson's meaning in saying that "the double-bind theory" is not so much a specific theory as a *language* (1)—which like any language serves to orient both thinking and observation.

From this standpoint, most of the writings that have aimed primarily at getting more simple and specific than the original article, especially those attempting to prove or disprove "the double-bind theory," miss the main point. This point is to consider and evaluate this communication more comprehensively— that is, like any communication, primarily by its effects. This is not to claim that care and precision in observation and statement—at a level appropriate to the situation—are not important, but that they are important functionally, not absolutely. It is certainly not to claim that evaluation of the article's significance on the basis of its effects is any simple matter. Such an evaluation requires many difficult judgements of the state of affairs before the communication, as its background; of its observable effects so far; even of estimated effects yet to come; and of the importance of any such changes and developments. I will not, in fact, venture to make any precise judgment in terms of this general standard. Broadly, however, against the background described earlier, I think it is plain that, despite any unclarities and confusions it included or led to, "Toward a Theory of Schizophrenia" did present a new general viewpoint on communication and behavior and the statement of this viewpoint has led to much other useful work, both practical and theoretical. In this connection, the various writings that have taken off from, and gone beyond, the original article (whether by expanding on matters merely touched on there or by seeking quite new connections) to consider other "pathologies," therapy, creativity, and even evolution do not appear as disqualifications. Rather, they represent developments consonant with the basic aims and framework of "Toward a Theory of Schizophrenia" and testify further to its usefulness and influence. And the end is not yet. To me, this seems the main thing, and enough.

## References

1. Bateson, G. (1966). "Slippery Theories," *International Journal of Psychiatry,* 2: 415-417.
2. Bateson, G., Jackson, D., Haley, J., & Weakland, J., (1956), "Toward a Theory of Schizophrenia," *Behavioral Science,* 1: 2.51-264, 1956.
3. Kuhn, T. (1962). *The Structure of Scientific Revolution,* Chicago, University of Chicago.
4. Olsen, D. (1972). "Empirically Unbinding the Double Bind: A Review of Research and Conceptual Reformulations," *Family Process,* 11: 69-94.

# CHAPTER 4

# Brief Therapy: Focused Problem Resolution[1]

*John H. Weakland, Richard Fisch, MD,*
*Paul Watzlawick, PhD,* and *Arthur M. Bodin, PhD*[2]

*This article describes a general view of the nature of human problems and their effective resolution and of related specific procedures, growing out of our prior work in family therapy, that have developed during six years of research on rapid problem resolution. With treatment limited to a maximum of ten sessions, we have achieved significant success in about three-fourths of a sample of 97 widely varied cases, and this approach to problems appears to have considerable potential for further development and wider application.*

In the last few years, brief treatment has been proliferating—both growing and dividing. As Barton's (1971) recent collection of papers illustrate, "Brief Therapy" means many different things to many different therapists. The brief therapy we wish to present here is an out-growth of our earlier work in that it

---

[1] Reprinted from *Family Process*, (13), 2, June, 141-168. The Brief Therapy Center was initiated by a grant from the Luke B. Hancock Foundation and matching funds from the T. B. Walker Foundation and the Robert C. Wheeler Foundation, whose support is gratefully acknowledged. In addition to the authors, the work of the Center has depended heavily on the services, largely volunteered, of Mrs. Barbara McLachlan as project secretary and of Mrs. Elaine Sorensen, Paul Druckman, MD, Frank D. Gerbode, M.D., Jack Simon, MD, Thomas M. Ferguson, Lynn Segal, George S. Greenberg, and Joel Latner as research assistants, at various periods.

We would also like to acknowledge the help of a number of guest therapists, whose work allowed us to observe and compare various treatment styles; these included Don D. Jackson, MD, Arthur B. Hardy, MD, Ralph I. Jacobs, MD, Roland C. Lowe, PhD, Patricia Hewitt, PhD, Constance Collinge Hansen, MSW, and Jay Haley, MA.

[2] Brief Therapy Center, Mental Research Institute, Palo Alto, California.

is based on two ideas central to family therapy: (a) focusing on observable behavioral interaction in the present and (b) deliberate intervention to alter the going system. In pursuing these themes further, however, we have arrived at a particular conceptualization of the nature of human problems and their effective resolution, and of related procedures, that is different from much current family therapy.

We have been developing and testing this approach at the Brief Therapy Center over the past six years. During this period the Center, operating one day a week, has treated 97 cases, in which 236 individuals were seen. (We have also had extensive experience using the same approach with private patients, but these cases have not been systematically followed up and evaluated.) These 97 cases reached us through a considerable variety of referral sources, and no deliberate selection was exercised. As a result, although probably a majority of our cases involve rather common marital and family problems, the sample covers a wide range overall. We have dealt with white, black, and oriental patients from 5 to over 60 years old, from welfare recipients to the very wealthy, and with a variety of both acute and chronic problems. These included school and work difficulties; identity crises; marital, family, and sexual problems; delinquency, alcohol, and eating problems; anxiety, depression, and schizophrenia. Regardless of the nature or severity of the problem, each case has been limited to a maximum of ten one-hour sessions, usually at weekly intervals. Under these circumstances, our treatment has been successful—in terms of achieving limited but significant goals related to the patients' main complaints—in about three-fourths of these cases. We have also demonstrated and taught our approach to a number of other therapists in our area.

We present our approach here for wider consideration. Any form of treatment, however, is difficult to convey adequately by a purely verbal account, without demonstration and direct observation. We will, therefore, begin by discussing the significance and nature of our basic premises in comparison with other forms of treatment. Hopefully, this will provide an orienting context for the subsequent description—supplemented with illustrative case material—of our interrelated concepts, plan of treatment, specific techniques, and results.

## Psychotherapy—Premises and Practices

In characterizing treatment approaches, although some over-simplification may result, outlining basic premises may make their nature—and especially, their implication—more plain. Often, attention is concentrated on what is explicit and detailed, while what is common and general is neglected. Yet, the more general an idea, the more determinative of behavior it is especially if its existence is not explicitly recognized. This holds for interpersonal influence as well as individual thinking and behavior; Robert Rosenthal's (1966) experiments demonstrate how the beliefs, assumptions, expectations, and biases of an experimenter or interviewer have a profound effect on his subjects. Similarly, the beliefs and theories held by a therapist may strongly influence not only his technique but also the length and outcome of his treatments—by affecting his patient's behavior, his evaluation of that behavior, or both.

For instance, if schizophrenia is conceptualized as a gradual, irreversible mental deterioration involving loss of contact with reality, then attempts at psychotherapeutic contact make little sense, and the only reasonable course of action is long-term hospitalization. The hospitalized patient is then likely to react in a way that clearly justifies this initial "preventive" action. Alternatively, if schizophrenia is seen as a manifestation of a dysfunctional structure of family relationships, the outlook is different and more hopeful, although basic restructuring of the family system is now likely to be seen as necessary. Again, in terms of the postulates of classical psychoanalytic theory, symptom removal must perforce lead to symptom displacement and exacerbation of the patient's condition, since it deals only with manifestations of deeper problems. The premises of the theory permit no other conclusion, except the alternative of claiming that the problem must not have been a "real" one (Saizman, 1968). On the other hand, in therapies based on learning or deconditioning theories, symptom manipulation is consistent with the theoretical premises. This enables the therapist to try very different intervention—and, to some extent, constrains him to do so.

That is, all theories of psychotherapy (including our own) have limitations, of practice as well as conception that are logically inherent in their own nature. Equally important, these limitations are often attributed to *human* nature, rather than to the nature of the theory. It is all too easy to overlook this and become enmeshed in unrecognized, circular explanations. Stating the basic premises of any psychotherapeutic theory as clearly and explicitly as possible at least helps toward perceiving also its implications, limitations, and possible alternatives.

## Our Brief Therapy—Cases and Comparisons

Much of the shorter-term treatment that has recently developed in response to the pressure of patient needs and situational limitations consists essentially of briefer versions of conventional forms of individual or family therapy. The same basic assumptions are involved, and, correspondingly, the methods used are similar, except for limited adaptations to the realities of fewer sessions (Barten & Barten, 1972; Bellak & Small, 1965; Rosenthal, 1970).

This is expectable, as the usual frameworks naturally offer more restraints to innovation than encouragement and guidance. Within their terms, new methods are apt to appear strange and unreliable (Krohn, 1971). Consequently, "brief therapy" ordinarily connotes an expedient that may be necessary when a preferred treatment is not available or is considered not feasible—since the "best" therapies often require patients equipped with rather exceptional resources of time, money, intelligence, persistence, and verbal sophistication. The goals of such brief therapy correspondingly are conceived as limited "first aid"—such as relief of some pressing but not fundamental aspect of the patient's problem, or a supportive holding action until really thorough treatment becomes possible.

We recognize and value the practical and economic advantages for patients and society of shortening treatment. We do not, however, see our own kind of brief treatment as an expedient, nor is brevity in itself a goal to us, except that we believe setting time limits on treatment has some positive influence on both therapists and patients. Rather the nature of our therapy, including its brevity, is primarily a consequence of our premises about the nature and handling of psychiatric problems.

Our fundamental premise is that regardless of their basic origins and etiology—if, indeed, these can ever be reliably determined—the kinds of problems people bring to psychotherapists *persist* only if they are maintained by on going current behavior of the patient and others with whom he interacts. Correspondingly, if such problem-maintaining behavior is appropriately changed or eliminated, the problem will be resolved or vanish, regardless of its nature, origin, or duration (Watzlawick, Beavin, & Jackson, 1967; Wender, 1968). Our general principles and specific practices of treatment all relate closely to these two assumptions.

This view, like any other, must be judged by its fruits rather than by its seeds. Yet, a brief consideration of two areas of shared prior experience and interest that appear to have had major implications for our present joint position may clarify it and give some due acknowledgement.

Our present brief therapy is visible first as pursuing further two main aspects of family therapy, in which we have all been extensively involved. A decade-and-a-half ago family therapy began to focus attention on observable behavioral interaction and its influence, both among family members and between them and the therapist, rather than on long-past events or inferred mental processes of individuals (Jackson, D., & Weakland, 1961). In line with this, we now see disturbed, deviant, or difficult behavior in an individual (like behavior generally) as essentially a social phenomenon, occurring as one aspect of a system, reflecting some dysfunction in that system, and best treated by some appropriate modification of that system. We differ, however, with those family therapists who consider the dysfunction involved to be necessarily a fundamental aspect of the system's organization and requiring correspondingly fundamental changes in the system. Instead, we now believe that apparently minor changes in overt behavior or its verbal labeling often are sufficient to initiate progressive developments. Further, while we recognize that along with its obvious disadvantages symptomatic behavior usually has some recognizable advantages or "pay-offs"—such as providing leverage in controlling relationships—we no longer consider these especially significant as causes of problems or obstacles to change.

Family therapy also has prompted greater activity by therapists. Once family interaction was seen as significant for problems, it followed that the therapist should aim to change the going system. Extending this, we now see the therapist's primary task as one of taking deliberate action to alter poorly functioning patterns of interaction as powerfully, effectively, and efficiently as possible.

On the matter of *how* the therapist can actively influence behavior effectively the strategy and techniques of change—we are especially indebted to the hypnotic work of Milton Erickson and his closely related psychotherapy.[3] Two points have been particularly influential.

First, although Erickson is much concerned with how overt behavior affects feelings or states of mind, his moves to change existing behavior usually depend upon implicit or indirect means of influence. Even when behavior is explicitly discussed, his aim often is not to clarify the "reality" of a situation but to alter and ameliorate it by some redefinition. Second, both as hypnotist and therapist, Erikson has emphasized the importance of "accepting what the client offers," and turning this to positive use—in ways we will illustrate later—even if what is "offered" might ordinarily appear as resistance or pathology.

While our present approach thus derives directly from basic family therapy, in part, and from Erickson's work, in part, it also differs from both. For example, many family therapists attempt to bring about change largely by explicit clarification of the nature of family behavior and interaction. Such an attempt now seems to us like a family version of promoting "insight," in which one tries to make clear to families the covert rules that have guided them; we ordinarily avoid this. Meanwhile, our conceptualization of problems and treatment appears at least more general and explicit than Erickson's and probably different in various specific respects.

---

[3] The work of Jay Haley (11, 12, 13) has been valuable in making Erickson's principles and practices more explicit, as well as in providing additional ideas from Haley's own work in family therapy and brief treatment.

On the other hand, similarities as well as differences are observable between our treatment approach and other approaches with which we have had little interaction. For example, within the general field of family therapy, we share with the crisis-intervention therapy of Pittman, Langsley, and their co-workers (1971), beliefs in the importance of situational change for the onset of problems and of both directive measures and negotiation of conflicts in promoting better functioning in family systems. Minuchin and Montalvo (1967), together with a number of their colleagues at the Philadelphia Child Guidance Clinic, have increasingly emphasized active intervention aimed at particular re-orderings of family relationship structure to achieve rapid problem resolution; we often pursue similar aims. Other family therapists than ourselves, notably Bowen, assign patients homework as part of treatment. Work with families similar to our own is also being developed abroad, for instance, at the Athenian Institute of Anthropos under Dr. George Vassiliou and at the Istituto per lo Studio della Famiglia in Milan, under Prof. Dr. Mara Selvini Palazzoli. In addition, the behavior modification school of therapy involves a number of ideas and interventions rather parallel to ours, although that field still appears to give little attention to systems of interaction. Furthermore, as noted later, a number of the techniques of intervention we utilize have also been used and described, though usually in a different conceptual context, by other therapists.

In sum, many particular conceptual and technical elements of our approach are not uniquely ours. We do, however, see as distinctive the overall system of explicitly stated and integrated ideas and practices that constitute our approach.

## Main Principles of Our Work

1. We are frankly symptom-oriented, in a broad sense. Patients or their family members come with certain complaints and accepting them for treatment involves a responsibility for relieving these complaints. Also, since deviant symptomatic behavior and its accompanying vicious circles of reaction and counter-reaction can themselves be so disruptive of system functioning, we believe that one should not hasten to seek other and deeper roots of pathology. The presenting problem offers, in one package, what the patient is ready to work on, a concentrated manifestation of whatever is wrong, and a concrete index of any progress made.

2. We view the problems that people bring to psychotherapists (except, of course, clearly organic psychiatric syndromes) as situational difficulties between people—problems of interaction. Most often this involves the identified patient and his family; however, other systems such as a patient's involvement

with others in a work situation may be important at times.

3. We regard such problems as primarily an outcome of everyday difficulties, usually involving adaptation to some life change that have been mishandled by the parties involved. When ordinary life difficulties are handled badly, unresolved problems tend increasingly to involve other life activities and relationships in impasses or crises, and symptom formation results.

4. While fortuitous life difficulties, such as illness, accidents, or loss of a job sometimes appear to initiate the development of a problem, we see normal transitional steps in family living as the most common and important "everyday difficulties" that may lead to problems. These transitions include: the change from the voluntary relationship of courtship to the commitment of marriage, and from this to the less reversible commitment when the first child is born; the sharing of influence with other authorities required when a child enters school, and with the child himself and his peers in the adolescent period; the shift from a child-oriented marital relationship back to a two-party system when the children leave the home, and its intensification at retirement; and return to single life at the death of one spouse. Although most people manage to handle these transitions at least passably well, they all require major changes in personal relationships that may readily be mishandled. This view is similar to that of Erickson and Haley (Haley, 1973).

5. We see two main ways by which "problems" are likely to develop: if people treat an ordinary difficulty as a "problem" or if they treat an ordinary (or worse) difficulty as no problem at all—that is, by either overemphasis or underemphasis of difficulties in living.

The first appears related to utopian expectations of life. There are countless difficulties which are part and parcel of the everyday business of living for which no known ideal or ultimate solutions exist. Even when relatively severe, these are manageable in themselves but can readily become "problems" as a result of a belief that there should or must be an ideal, ultimate solution for them. For instance, there apparently has been a "generation gap" for the past 5000 years that we know of, but its difficulties only became greatly exacerbated into a "problem" when many people became convinced that it should be closed.

Inversely, but equally, "problems" can arise out of the denial of manifest difficulties—which could be seen as utopian assertions. For instance, the husband and wife who insist their marriage was made in heaven, or the parents who deny the existence of any conflicts with their children—and who may contend that any one seeing any difficulty must be either bad or mad—are likely to be laying the foundation for some outbreak of symptomatic behavior.

Two other aspects of this matter need mention. First, over-or under-emphasis of life difficulties is not entirely a matter of personal or family characteristics; this depends also on more general cultural attitudes and conceptions. While these often may be helpful in defining and dealing with the common vicissitudes of social life, they can also be unrealistic and provoke problems. For example, except for the death of a spouse, our own culture characterizes most of the transitions listed earlier as wonderful steps forward along life's path. Since all of these steps ordinarily involve significant and inescapable difficulties, such over-optimistic characterization increases the likelihood of problems developing—especially for people who take what they are told seriously. Second, inappropriate evaluation and handling of difficult situations is often multiplied by interaction between various parties involved. If two persons have similar inappropriate views, they may reciprocally reinforce their common error, while if one over-emphasizes a difficulty and another under-emphasizes it, interaction may lead to increasing polarization and an even more inappropriate stance by each.

6. We assume that once a difficulty begins to be seen as a "problem," the continuation, and often the exacerbation, of this problem results from the creation of a positive feedback loop, most often centering around those very behaviors of the individuals in the system that are intended to resolve the difficulty: The original difficulty is met with an attempted "solution" that intensifies the original difficulty, and so on and on (Wender, 1968).

Consider, for instance, a common pattern between a depressed patient and his family. The more they try to cheer him up and make him see the positive sides of life, the more depressed the patient is likely to get: "They don't even understand me." The action meant to *alleviate* the behavior of the other party *aggravates* it; the "cure" becomes worse than the original "disease." Unfortunately, this usually remains unnoted by those involved and even is disbelieved if any one else tries to point it out.

7. We view long-standing problems or symptoms not as "chronicity" in the usual implication of some basic defect in the individual or family, nor even that a problem has become "set" over time, but as the persistence of a *repetitively* poorly handled difficulty. People with chronic problems have just been struggling inappropriately for longer periods of time. We, therefore, assume that chronic problems offer as great an opportunity for change as acute problems and that the principal difference lies in the usually pessimistic expectations of therapists facing a chronic situation.

8. We see the resolution of problems as primarily requiring a substitution of behavior patterns so as to interrupt the vicious, positive feedback circles. Other less destructive and less distressing behaviors are potentially open to the patient and involved family members at all times. It is usually impossible, however, for them to change from their rigidly patterned, traditional, unsuccessful problem-solving behavior to more appropriate behavior on their own initiative. This is especially likely when such usual behavior is culturally supported, as is often the case: Everyone *knows* that people should do their best to encourage and cheer up a loved one who is sad and depressed. Such behavior is both "right" and "logical"—but often it just doesn't work.

9. In contrast, we seek means of promoting beneficial change that works, even if our remedies appear illogical. For instance, we would be likely to comment on how sad a depressed patient looks and to suggest that there must be some real and important reason for this. Once given some information on the situation, we might say it is rather strange that he is not even *more* depressed. The usual result, paradoxical as it may seem, is that the patient begins to look and sound better.

10. In addition to accepting what the patient offers, and reversing the usual "treatment" that has served to make matters worse, this simple example also illustrates our concept of "thinking small" by focusing on the symptom presented and working in a limited way towards its relief.

We contend generally that change can be effected most easily if the goal of change is reasonably small and clearly stated. Once the patient has experienced a small but definite change in the seemingly monolithic nature of the problem most real to him, the experience leads to further, self-induced changes in this, and often also, in other areas of his life. That is, beneficent circles are initiated.

This view may seem insensitive to the "real," "big," or "basic" problems that many therapists and patients expect to be changed by therapy. Such goals are often vague or unrealistic, however, so that therapy which is very optimistic in concept easily becomes lengthy and disappointing in actual practice. Views of human problems that are either pessimistic about change or grandiose about the degree of change needed undermine the therapist's potentially powerful influence for limited but significant change.

11. Our approach is fundamentally pragmatic. We try to base our conceptions and our interventions on direct observation in the treatment situation of *what* is going on in systems of human interaction, *how* they continue to function in such ways, and *how* they may be altered most effectively.

Correspondingly, we avoid the question "Why?" From our standpoint, this question is not relevant, and involvement with it commonly leads toward concerns about "deeper" underlying causes—historical, mental, familial—of problem behavior and about "insight" into these.

That is, the question "Why?" tends to promote an individualistic, voluntaristic, and rationalistic conception of human behavior, rather than one focused on systems of interaction and influence. Moreover, since underlying causes inherently are inferential rather than observable, concern about them distracts a therapist from close observation of the present problem and what behavior may be perpetuating it.

On the basis of this general conception of problems and their resolution, which is discussed more fully in Watzlawick, Weakland, and Fisch (1974), we can now describe the overall practical approach and specific techniques that we utilize.

## Operation of the Brief Therapy Center

The Brief Therapy Center was established as one of the projects at the Mental Research Institute in January, 1967. Since the termination of our founding grants, we have continued our work on a somewhat reduced scale on volunteered time. Some direct operating expenses have been met by donations from patients, although we provide free treatment where appropriate.

Our working quarters consist of a treatment room and observation room, separated by a one-way viewing screen, with provision for simultaneously listening to and tape-recording sessions. There is also an intercom phone between the two rooms. At the outset of our work, a therapist and an official observer were assigned, in rotation, to each case. More recently, we have been working as an overall team, with several observers of equal status usually present.

Our handling of all cases follows a six-stage schema, although in practice there may be some overlap among these:
1. Introduction to our treatment set-up.
2. Inquiry and definition of the problem.
3. Estimation of behavior maintaining the problem.
4. Setting goals of treatment.
5. Selecting and making behavioral interventions.
6. Termination.
Each of these will now be considered in order.

## Introduction to Our Treatment & Set-Up

Patients intentionally are accepted with no screening. A first appointment is set by the project secretary whenever an applicant calls and there is a vacancy in our schedule. No waiting lists are kept; when we have no vacancy, people are referred elsewhere.

At the first meeting, our secretary has the patient or family fill out a form covering basic demographic data and brings him or them to the treatment room. The therapist begins by explaining the physical and organizational arrangements, mentioning the potential advantages for treatment of the recording and observation, and requests written consent to this. Only two patients have ever declined to proceed on this basis. The therapist also tells the patient at once that we work on a maximum of ten sessions per case; this helps to set a positive expectation of rapid change.

## Definition of the Problem

Since our treatment focus is symptomatic, we want first to get a clear and explicit statement of the presenting complaint. Therefore, as soon as the therapist has taken a brief record of the referral source and any previous treatment, he asks what problem has brought the patient to see us. If a patient states a number of complaints, we will ask which is the most important. In marital or family cases, since viewpoints may differ, although they often are plainly interrelated, we ask each of the parties involved to state his own main complaint. From the beginning, then, we are following a form of the general principle, "Start where the patient is at."

Fairly often, the patient will give an adequate answer—by which we mean a clear statement referring to concrete behavior. In many cases, however, the response will leave the presenting problem still in doubt. Further inquiry is then needed to define more clearly this point of departure for the entire treatment. For example, patients with previous treatment experience or psychological sophistication are likely, after only the briefest mention of any present behavioral difficulty, to launch into discussion of presumed underlying matters, especially intrapsychic factors and family history, presenting these as the "real problem." We then press the question of what particular difficulties in living have brought them to see us *now.* To make things more specific, we often ask such questions as "What do you now do because of your problem that you want to stop doing, or do differently?" and "What would you like to do that your problem interferes with doing now?" Such inquiries also begin to raise the related question of treatment goals.

Other patients, especially younger ones, may state their complaints in vague terms that lack reference to any concrete behavior or life situation: "I don't know who I really am" or "We just can't communicate." Such patients can be particularly difficult initially. We find it important not to accept such statements as appropriate and informative but to continue inquiry until at least the therapist, if not the patient, can formulate a concrete, behavioral picture of the problem—of which such attachment to vague and often grandiose thinking and talking may itself be a major aspect.

## Estimation of Behavior Maintaining the Problem

Our view, as mentioned earlier, is that problem behavior persists only when it is repeatedly reinforced in the course of social interaction between the patient and other significant people. Usually, moreover, it is just what the patient and these others are doing in their efforts to deal with the problem—often those attempts at help that appear most "logical" or unquestionably right—that is most important in maintaining or exacerbating it.

Once behavior is observed and considered in this light, the way this occurs is often rather obvious: The wife who nags her husband and hides his bottle in her efforts to save him from his alcohol problem and succeeds only in continually keeping drinking uppermost in his mind; the forgiving husband who never criticizes his wife until she feels he doesn't care anything about her, whatever she does, and becomes depressed—and he is forgiving of that too; the parents of a child dissatisfied with school who "encourage" him by talking all the more about how important and great education is—instead of it being a necessary drag. In other instances, of course, the reinforcements may be more difficult to perceive, either because they are subtle or complex—nonverbal behaviors, contradictions between statements and actions, different behaviors by several persons—or because even therapists are conditioned to accept cultural standards of logic and rightness without examining whether things really work that way.

In practice, the therapist first simply asks the patient and any family members present how they have been trying to deal with the problem. This alone may lead rapidly to a view of what keeps things going badly. If not, the inquiry, aiming always at concrete behavior, can be pursued at more length and in more detail, but sympathetically—the therapist's aim is to get enough information to understand what is happening, for which he needs cooperation, not to confront people with their mistakes. In addition to what the patient or others state explicitly, it is important to note *how* they discuss the problem and its handling, including their interaction. Such inquiry is likely to disclose a number of things that play some part in maintaining the problem, but working briefly demands choosing priorities. On the basis of observation and experience, one must judge which behavior seems most crucial.

## Setting Goals of Treatment

Setting a goal both acts as a positive suggestion that change is feasible in the time allotted and provides a criterion of therapeutic accomplishment for therapist and patient. We, therefore, want goals stated clearly in terms of observable, concrete behavior to minimize any possibility of uncertainty or denial later. If parents bring us a child because he is failing in school, we ask for an explicit criterion of satisfactory progress—because we want to avoid subsequent equivocations such as "He is getting B's now instead of F's, but he isn't really learning enough." Also, we steer toward "thinking small" for reasons already discussed. Therefore, our usual inquiry is something like "At a minimum, what (change in) behavior would indicate to you that a definite step forward has been made on your problem?"

Concerning goals especially, however, patients often talk in vague or sweeping terms, despite our efforts to frame the question in terms of specific behavior. We then try to get more concrete answers by further discussion, clarification, and presentation of examples of possible goals for consideration. With vague, grandiose, or utopian patients, we have found it helpful to reverse our field, bringing them down to earth by suggesting goals that are too far out even for them. This again involves accepting what the patient offers, and even enlarging on this, in order to change it. For example, a student who was already in his mid-20's and was still being supported by a working mother told us he was studying "philosophical anthropology" in order to bring the light of India and China to bear on the West. He also, however, mentioned some interest in attending a well-known school of Indian music. It was then pointed out to him that this represented a rather limited aim compared to his concern to unite the spirituality of India with the practical communism of China and use both to reconstruct Western society. He then said that, since he was not doing well in his studies and was short of money, if he could secure a scholarship and really learn Indian music, this would be quite enough accomplishment for the present.

We usually are able, directly or indirectly, to obtain a stated goal that appears sufficiently explicit and appropriate to the problem. In some cases, however, we have not been able to do so. Either the patient persisted in stating only vague, untestable goals, or, rarely, the patient stated and stuck to an explicit goal which we judged inappropriate to his problem. Then we do not dispute what the patient insists on but privately set our own goal for the case by joint staff discussion of what sort of behavior would best exemplify positive change for the particular patient and problem. In fact, some such discussion occurs for all cases; at the least, the staff must always judge whether the patient's statement of his goal is adequate. Also, there is always staff discussion of intermediate behavioral goals; how does the patient or his family member need to behave so that the specific goal of treatment will follow?[4]

Our aim is to have a definite goal established by the second session, but gathering and digesting the information needed for this sometimes takes longer. Occasionally, we may revise the original goal in the course of treatment or add a secondary goal.

## Selecting and Making Interventions

Once we have formed a picture of current behavior central to the problem and estimated what different behavior would lead to the specific goal selected, the task is one of intervening to promote such change. This stage must be discussed at some length, since it ordinarily constitutes the largest, most varied, and probably most unusual part of our treatment.

*Change and "insight."* We have already stated that our aim is to produce behavior change and that we do not see working toward insight, at either an individual or a family level, as of much use in this. In fact, working toward insight can even be counter-productive. Simple, practical-minded patients are often put off by this, since they want action and results, while more intellectually minded patients are likely to welcome such an approach but use it to delay or defeat any change in actual behavior. However, in addition to suggesting or prescribing changes in overt behavior, we do utilize interpretations. Our aim, though, is simply the useful relabeling of behavior. Patients often interpret their own behavior, or that of others, in ways that make for continuing difficulties. If we can only redefine the meaning or implications attributed to the behavior, this itself may have a powerful effect on attitudes, responses and relationships. Such interpretation might look like an attempt to impart insight, but it is not. Using interpretation to promote insight implies that truth can helpfully be disclosed and recognized. This is not our aim or our belief. Rather, our view is that redefining behavior labeled "hostile" as "concerned interest," for example, may be therapeutically useful whether or not *either* label is "true," and that such truth can never be firmly established. All that is observable is that some labels provoke difficulties, while others, achievable by redefinition, promote adjustment and harmony—but this is enough.

Such relabeling may be especially important with rigid patients. It does not require overt behavior change, and it may even be accomplished without the need for *any* active cooperation by the patient or any family member. If the

---

[4] Our schedule is arranged to allow for one half-hour after each session for staff discussion and planning of goals, specific interventions to use, and so on. In addition, new caees and general issues are considered at more length in separate, weekly staff meetings.

therapist's redefinition of an action or situation is not openly challenged—which can usually be arranged—then the meaning and effects of that behavior have already been altered.

*Use of idiosyncratic characteristics and motivation.* We attempt early in treatment to determine what approach would appeal most to the particular patient—to observe "where he lives" and meet this need, whether it is to believe in the magical, to defeat the expert, to be a caretaker of someone, to face a challenge, or whatever. Since the consequences of any such characteristic depend greatly on the situation in which it operates and how this is defined, we see these characteristics of different individuals not as obstacles or deficiencies, but as potential levers for useful interventions by the therapist.

For example, certain patients appear inclined toward defeating therapists, despite their request for help. This may be indicated by a history of unsuccessful treatment, repeated failure to understand explanations or carry out instructions, and so on. In such cases, the easiest and most effective course may be for the therapist to insist that the patient cannot possibly resolve his problem and that treatment can at most help him to endure it better. The patient is then likely to defeat *this* stance by improving.

A middle-aged widow first came to us with a complaint about the behavior of her 18-year-old son: delinquency, school failures, anger, and threatened violence toward her. She stated this was her only problem, although she also mentioned that she was an epileptic and was unable to use her right arm as a result of a work injury. Both mother and son had had about two years of previous therapy. We first suggested directly that her son was acting like a difficult, provoking, overgrown kid and, accordingly, what she might gain by handling him more firmly in a few simple ways. She quickly thwarted such suggestions by increasing claims of helplessness: now the epilepsy was emphasized; there was trouble with the other arm, too; a hysterectomy and appendectomy were also reported, along with childhood rheumatic fever, bleeding gums, troubles with her former husband and with her mother-in-law, constant worsening financial crises, and much more. In short, she was already a woman carrying on bravely amidst a sea of troubles that would have totally swamped anyone else; how could we ask her to do more yet? We then changed our approach to utilize this characteristic opposition. We began to insist to her that she was being unduly optimistic, was minimizing her troubles in an unrealistic way, and was not recognizing that the future very probably held even greater disasters for her, both individually and in terms of her son's behavior. It took some doing to surpass her own pessimistic line, but once we were able to do so, she began to improve. She started to oppose our pessimism—which she could only do by claiming and proving that she was not *that* sick and helpless—and to take a much more assertive attitude with her son, to which he responded well.

*Directed behavior change.* One of our main stated aims is to change overt behavior—to get people to stop doing things that maintain the problem and to do others that will lead toward the goal of treatment. While we are willing to issue authoritative directions, we find compliant patients rather rare. After all, most patients have already been exposed to lots of advice. If it was good, they must have some difficulty about profiting from advice; if it was bad, some preparation is needed for them to respond to quite different advice. Moreover, again, it is often just that behavior that seems most logical to people that is perpetuating their problems. They then need special help to do what will seem illogical and mistaken. When sitting on a nervous horse, it is not easy to follow the instructor's orders to let go of the reins. One *knows* the horse will run away, even though it is really the pull on the reins that is making him jump.

Behavioral instructions therefore are more effective when carefully framed and made indirect, implicit, or apparently insignificant. When requesting changes, it is helpful to minimize either the matter or the manner of the request. We will suggest a change rather than order it. If the patient still appears reluctant, we will back off further. We may then suggest it is too early to do that thing; the patient might think about it but be sure not to take any action yet. When we do request particular actions, we may ask that they be done once or twice at most before we meet again. We may request only actions that will appear minor to the patient, although in our view they represent the first in a series of steps, or involve a microcosm of the central difficulty. For example, a patient who avoids making any demands of others in his personal relationships may be assigned the task of asking for one gallon of gasoline at a service station, specifically requesting each of the usual free services, and offering a twenty-dollar bill in payment.

This example also illustrates our use of "homework" assignments to be carried out between sessions. Homework of various kinds is regularly employed, both to utilize time more fully and to promote positive change where it counts most, in real life outside the treatment room.

*Paradoxical instructions.* Most generally, paradoxical instruction involves prescribing behavior that appears in opposition to the goals being sought, in order actually to move toward them. This may be seen as an inverse to pursuing "logical" courses that lead only to more trouble. Such instructions probably constitute the most important single class of interventions in our treatment. This technique is not new; aspects and examples of it have been described by Frankl (1957, 1960), Haley (1963), Newton (1968) and Watzlawick, et al. (1967). We have simply related this technique to our overall approach and elaborated on its use.

Paradoxical instruction is used most frequently in the form of case-specific "symptom prescription," the apparent encouragement of symptomatic or other undesirable behavior in order to lessen such behavior or bring it under control. For example, a patient who complains of a circumscribed, physical symptom—headache, insomnia, nervous mannerisms, or whatever—may be told that during the coming week, usually for specified periods, he should make every effort to increase the symptom. A motivating explanation usually is given, e.g., that if he can succeed in making it worse, he will at least suffer less from a feeling of helpless lack of control. Acting on such a prescription usually results in a *decrease* of the symptom—which is desirable. But even if the patient makes the symptom increase, this too is good. He has followed the therapist's instruction, and the result has shown that the apparently unchangeable problem can change. Patients often present therapists with impossible-looking problems, to which every possible response seems a poor one. It is comforting, in turn, to be able to offer the patient a "therapeutic double bind" (Bateson et. al, 1956), which promotes progress no matter which alternative response he makes.

The same approach applies equally to problems of interaction. When a schizophrenic son used bizarre, verbal behavior to paralyze appropriate action by his parents, we suggested that when he needed to defend himself against the parents' demands, he could intimidate them by acting crazy. Since this instruction was given in the parents' presence, there were two paradoxical positive effects: the son decreased his bizarreness and the parents became less anxious and paralyzed by any such behavior.

Not infrequently, colleagues find it hard to believe that patients will really accept such outlandish prescriptions, but they usually do so readily. In the first place, the therapist occupies a position of advice-giving expert. Second, he takes care to frame his prescriptions in a way most likely to be accepted, from giving a rationale appropriate to the particular patient to refusing any rationale on the grounds that the patient needs to discover somethings quite unanticipated. Third, we often are really just asking the patient to do things they already are doing, only on a different basis.

We may also encourage patients to use similar paradoxes themselves, particularly with spouses or children. Thus, a parent concerned about her child's poor school homework (but who probably was covertly discouraging him) was asked to teach the child more self-reliance by offering incorrect answers to the problems he was asking help in solving.

Paradoxical instructions at a more general level are often used also. For example, in direct contrast to our name and ten-session limit, we almost routinely stress "going slow" to our patients at the outset of treatment and, later, by greeting a patient's report of improvement with a worried look and the statement, "I think things are moving a bit too fast." We also do the same thing more implicitly, by our emphasis on minimal goals, or by pointing out possible disadvantages of improvement to patients, "You would like to do much better at work, but are you prepared to handle the problem of envy by your colleagues?" Such warnings paradoxically promote rapid improvement, apparently by reducing any anxiety about change and increasing the patient's desire to get on with things to counteract the therapist's apparent over cautiousness.

On the same principle, when a patient shows unusually rapid or dramatic improvement, after acknowledging this change we may prescribe a relapse, on the rationale that it further increases control: "Now you have managed to turn the symptom off. If you can manage to turning it back on during this next week, you will have achieved even more control over it." This intervention, similar to Rosen's "re-enacting the psychosis" (Pitman et. al., 1971) and related techniques of Erickson, anticipates that in some patients improvement may increase apprehension about change and meets this danger by paradoxically redefining any relapse that might occur as a step forward rather than backward.

Since we as therapists are by definition experts, giving authoritative instructions on both thinking and acting, another pervasive element of paradox is created by the fact that ordinarily we do so only tentatively, by suggestions or questions rather than direct orders, and often adopt a "one-down" position of apparent ignorance or confusion. We find that patients, like other people, accept and follow advice more readily when we avoid "coming on strong."

***Utilization of interpersonal influence.*** Although many of our treatment sessions include directly only one therapist and one patient, we consider and utilize more extended interpersonal relationships constantly in our work. First, even when we see only the "identified patient," we conceive the problem in terms of some system of relationships and problem-maintaining behavior involving his family, his friends, or his work situation. Therefore, we believe that any interventions made with the patient must also take their probable consequences for others into account. Equally, however, useful interventions may be made at any point in the system, and frequently it appears more effective to focus our efforts on someone other than the identified patient. Where a child is the locus of the presenting problem, we very commonly see the whole family only once or twice. After this we see the parents only and work with them on modifying their handling of the child or their own interaction. With couples also, we may see the spouses separately for the most part, often spending more time with the one seen by them as "normal." Our point is that effective inter-vention anywhere in a system produces changes throughout, but according to what the situation offers, one person or another may be more accessible to us, more open to influence, or a better lever for change in the system.

Second, the therapist and the observers also constitute a system of relation-ships that is frequently used to facilitate treatment. With patients who find it difficult to accept advice directly from a real live person, an observer may make comments to the therapist over the intercom phone to be relayed to the patient from this unseen and presumably objective authority. When a patient tends to disagree constantly, an observer may enter and criticize the therapist for his "poor understanding" of the case, forming an apparent alliance with the patient. The observer can then often successfully convey re-phrased ver-sions of what the therapist was offering originally. With patients who alternate between two different stances, two members of the treatment team may agree, separately, with the two positions. Then, whatever course the patient takes next he is going along with a therapist's interpretation, and further suggestions can be given and accepted more successfully. Such therapist-observer interac-tion strategies can bring about change rapidly even with supposedly "difficult" patients.

As may be evident, all of these techniques of intervention are means to-ward maximizing the range and power of the therapist's influence. Some will certainly see, and perhaps reject, such interventions as manipulative. Rather than arguing over this, we will simply state our basic view. First, influence is an inherent element in all human contact. Second, the therapist's functioning nec-essarily includes this fact of life, but goes much further; professionally he is a specialist at influence. People come to a therapist because they are not satisfied with some aspect of their living, have been unable to change it, and are seeking help in this. In taking any case, therefore, the therapist accepts the assignment of influencing people's behavior, feelings, or ideas toward desirable ends. Ac-cordingly, third, the primary responsibility of the therapist is to seek out and apply appropriate and effective means of influence. Of course, this includes taking full account of the patient's stated and observed situation and aims. Given these, though, the therapist still must make choices of what to say and do, and equally what not to say and do. This inherent responsibility cannot be escaped by following some standard method of treatment regardless of its re-sults, by simply following the patient's lead, or even by following a moral ideal of always being straightforward and open with the patient. Such courses, even if possible, themselves represent strategic choices. To us, the most fundamen-tal point is whether the therapist attempts to deny the necessity of such choices to himself, not what he tells the patient about them. We believe the better course is to recognize this necessity.

Team work facilitates such interventions but actually is seldom essential. A single therapist who is flexible and not unduly concerned about being correct and consistent can also utilize similar technique—for example, by stating two different positions himself to try whatever means of influence are judged most promising in the circumstances, and to accept responsibility for the consequences.

*Termination.* Whether cases run the limit of ten sessions or goals are achieved sooner, we usually briefly review the course of treatment with the patient, pointing out any apparent gains—giving the patient maximum credit for this achievement and noting any matters unresolved. We also remark on the probable future beyond termination, ordinarily in connection with reminding patients that we will be contacting them for a follow-up interview in about three months. This discussion usually embodies positive suggestions about further improvement. We may remind patients that our treatment was not intended to achieve final solutions, but an initial breakthrough on which they themselves can build further. In a minority of cases, however—particularly with negativistic patients, ones who have difficulty acknowledging help from anyone, or those fond of challenges—we may take an opposite tack, minimizing any positive results of treatment and expressing skepticism about any progress in the future. In both instances, our aim is the same, to extend our therapeutic influence beyond the period of actual contact.

In some cases, we encounter patients who make progress but seem unsure of this and concerned about termination. We often meet this problem by means of terminating without termination. That is, we say we think enough has been accomplished to terminate, but this is not certain; it can really be judged only by how actual life experience goes over a period of time. Therefore, we propose to halt treatment, but to keep any remainder of the ten sessions "in the bank," available to draw on if the patient should encounter some special difficulty later. Usually, the patient then departs more at ease and does not call upon us further.

## Evaluation and Results

If psychotherapy is to be taken seriously as treatment, not just an interesting exploratory or expressive experience, its effectiveness must be reliably evaluated. But this is far from easy, and rather commonly therapists offer only general clinical impressions of their results, with no follow-up of cases after termination, while researchers present ideal study designs that seldom get implemented.

We certainly cannot claim to have resolved this problem fully, even though we have been concerned with systematic evaluation of results from the outset of our work. Our method of evaluation still involves some clinical judgments and occasional ambiguities, despite efforts to minimize these. Until very recently, we have not had the resources needed to repeat our short-term follow-ups systematically after longer periods. And our evaluation plan is apt to seem overly simple in comparison with such comprehensive schemes as that of Fiske, et al. (Fiske, Hunt, Luborsky, Orne, Parloff, Reiser, & Tuma, 1970). At most, we can claim only that our method of evaluation is simple, avoiding dependence upon either elaborate manipulation and interpretation of masses of detailed data or elaborate theoretical inference; that it is reasonably systematic and practicable; and most important, that it is consonant with our overall approach to problems and treatment.

We see the essential task of evaluation as systematic comparison of what treatment *proposes* to do and its observable *results.* Our treatment aim is to change patients' behavior in specific respects, in order to resolve the main presenting complaint. Given the brevity of our work, the past refractoriness of most of the problems presented, and our frequent observation of behavior change immediately following particular interventions, we feel fairly safe in crediting observed changes to our treatment. Our evaluation then depends on answers to the two questions: Has behavior changed as planned?  Has the complaint been relieved?

In our follow-up, the interviewer, who has not participated in the treatment, first inquires whether the specified treatment goal has been met. For instance, "Are you still living with your mother, or are you living in your own quarters now?" Next, the patient is asked the current status of the main complaint. This is supplemented by inquiring whether any further therapy has been sought since terminating with us. The patient is also asked whether any improvements have occurred in areas not specifically dealt with in treatment. Finally, to check on the supposed danger of symptom substitution, the patient is routinely asked if any new problems have appeared.

Ideally, such evaluation would divide our cases into two neat piles:  successes in which our goal of behavior change was met and the patient's problem completely resolved, and failures in both respects. In reality, our treatment is not perfect; while results in these terms are clear for a majority of cases, several sources of less clear-cut outcomes remain: (a) Fairly often we have had cases in which our goal was reached or approached and considerable improvement was evident, but complete resolution of the presenting problem or problems was not attained. (b) Occasionally we have failed to formulate a goal explicit and concrete enough to check on its achievement with certainty. (c)  In a very few cases, achievement of the planned goal and reported relief of the problem have been inversely related—hitting our target of change did not lead to relief, or we somehow got results in spite of missing our specific target.

In terms of our basic principles, all such mixed eases must be considered as failures of either conception or execution that demand further study. In the patients' terms, on the other hand, some of these cases have been completely successful, and many others represent quite significant progress. For the more limited and immediate purpose of evaluating the general utility of our approach, therefore, we have classified our cases into three groups according to practical results, recognizing that these correlate generally but not completely with achievement of our specific goals of behavior change. These groups represent: (a) complete relief of the presenting complaint; (b) clear and considerable, but not complete, relief of the complaint; and (c) little or no such change. For simplicity, the one case in which things were worse after treatment is included in the third group. We have not broken down our sample into subgroups based on common diagnosis, since the conventional system of diagnostic categories and our conception of problems and their treatment are based on different assumptions and the nature of the presenting problem has appeared to make little difference for our rate of success or failure. It should also be noted that this evaluation refers directly only to the major presenting complaint. However, in none of our cases in which this complaint was resolved was there any report of new problems arising, and in many of these improvements in additional areas were reported. On this basis, then, our overall results for 97 cases, involving an average of 7.0 sessions, are:

| | | |
|---|---|---|
| Success | 39 cases | 40 per cent |
| Significant improvement | 31 cases | 32 per cent |
| Failure | 27 cases | 28 per cent |

These results appear generally comparable to those reported for various forms of longer-term treatment.

## Conclusion: Implications

In this paper we have set forth a particular conception of the nature of psychiatric problems, described a corresponding brief treatment approach and techniques, and presented some results of their application. Clearly, further clinical research should be done, as important problems obviously remain; goals are still difficult to set in certain types of cases, the choice of interventions has not been systematized, evaluation is not perfected. Concurrently, though, there should also be more thinking about the broader significance of these ideas and methods. Our results already give considerable evidence for the usefulness of our general conception of human problems and their practical handling. Since this is both quite different from more common views and potentially widely relevant, we will conclude with a tentative consideration of some broad implications of our work.

The most immediate and evident potential of our work is for more effective use of existing psychiatric facilities and personnel. This could include reduction in the usual length of treatment and a corresponding increase in the number of patients treated, with no sacrifice of effectiveness. In fact, our approach gives promise of more than ordinary effectiveness with a variety of common but refractory problems, such as character disorders, marital difficulties, psychoses, and chronic problems generally. Further, it is not restricted to highly educated and articulate middle-class patients but is applicable to patients of whatever class and educational background.

In addition, our approach is relatively clear and simple. It might therefore be feasible to teach its effective use to considerable numbers of lay therapists. Even if some continuing supervision from professionals should be necessary, the combination of brief treatment and many therapists thus made possible could help greatly in meeting present needs for psychological help. Although this kind of development would have little to offer private practice, it could be significant for the work of overburdened social agencies.

Taking a wider view, it is also important that our model sees behavioral difficulties "all under one roof" in two respects. First, our model interrelates individual behavior and its social context instead of dividing them—not only within the family, but potentially at all levels of social organization. Second, this framework helps to identify continuities, similarities, and interrelations between normal everyday problems, psychiatric problems of deviant individual behavior, and many sorts of socially problematic behavior, such as crime, social isolation and anomie, and certain aspects of failure and poverty. At present, social agencies attempting to deal with such problems at the individual or family level are characterized by marked conceptual and organizational divisions—between psychological vs. sociological, supportive vs. disciplinary orientations, and more specifically, in the division of problems into many categories that are presumed to be distinct and discrete—reminiscent of the "syndromes" of conventional psychiatry. At best, this results in discontinuity; ineffective, partial approaches; or reduplication of efforts. At worst, it appears increasingly likely that such divisions themselves may function to reinforce inappropriate attempts at solution of many kinds of problems, as suggested by Auerswald (1968) and Hoffman and Long (1969). Our work thus suggests a need and a potential basis for a more unified and effective organization of social services.

Finally, our work has still broader implications that deserve explicit recognition, even though any implementation necessarily would be a very long-range and difficult problem. Our theoretical viewpoint is focused on the ways in which problems of behavior and their resolution are related to social interaction. Such problems occur not only with individuals and families, but also at every wider level of social organization and functioning. We can already discern two kinds of parallels between problems met in our clinical work and larger social problems. Problems may be reduplicated widely, as when concern about differences between parents and children becomes, in the large, "the generation gap problem." And conflicts between groups—whether these groups are economic, racial, or political—may parallel those seen between individuals. Our work, like much recent social history, suggests very strongly that ordinary, "common-sense" ways of dealing with such problems often fail, and, indeed, often exacerbate the difficulty. Correspondingly, some of our uncommon ideas and techniques for problem-resolution might eventually be adapted for application to such wider spheres of human behavior.

## References

Auerswald, E. (1968). Interdisciplinary vs. Ecological Approach, *Family Process*, 7: 202-215.

Barten, H. (Ed.) (1971). *Brief Therapies*, New York, Behavioral Publications.

Barten, H., & Barten, S., (Eds.), (1972). *Children & Their Parents in Brief Therapy*, New York, Behavioral Publications.

Bateson, G., Jackson, D., Haley, J., & Weakland, J. (1956). Toward a Theory of Schizophrenia, *Behavioral Science*, 1 (1) : 251-264.

Bellak, L., & Small, L. (1965). *Emergency Psychotherapy & Brief Psychotherapy*, New York, Grune & Stratton.

Fiske, D., Hunt, H., Luborsky, L., Orne, M., Parloff, M., Reiser, M., & Tuma, A. (1970). Research on Effectiveness of Psychotherapy, *Archives of General Psychiatry*, 22: 22-32.

Frank, J. (1961). *Persuasion & Healing*, Baltimore, Johns Hopkins Press.

Frankl, V. (1957). *The Doctor & the Soul*, New York, Alfred A. Knopf

Frankl, V. (1960). Paradoxical Interventions, *Am. Journal of Psychotherapy*, 14: 52-535.

Jackson, D., & Weakland, J. (1961).Conjoint Family Therapy: Some Considerations on Theory, Technique, and Results, *Psychiatry*, Supplement to 24:2: 3045.

Haley, J. (1963). *Strategies of Psychotherapy*, New York, Grune and Stratton.

Haley, J. (1973). *Uncommon Therapy: The Psychiatric Techniques of Milton H. Erickson, M.D.*, New York, W. W. Norton.

Haley, J. (Ed.) (1969). *Advanced Techniques of Hypnosis and Therapy: Selected Papers of Milton H. Erickson, M.D.*, New York, Grune and Stratton.

Hoffman, L., & Long, L., (1969). A Systems Dilemma, *Family Process*, 8: 211-234.

Krohn, A. (1971). Beyond Interpretation, (A review of M.D. Nelson, et al., "Roles and Paradigms in Psychotherapy"). *Contemporary Psychology*, 16: 38 -382.

Minuchin, S., & Montalvo, B. (1967). Techniques for working with disorganized low socioeconomic families, *American Journal of Orthopsychiatry*, 37: 88-7.

Newton, J. (1968). Considerations for the Psychotherapeutic Technique of Symptom Scheduling, *Psychotherapy: Theory, Research & Practice*, 5: 9-103.

Pittman, F, Langsley, D., Flomenhaft, K., De Young, C., Machotka, P., & Kaplan, D., (1971). Therapy Techniques of the Family Treatment Unit, pp. 25-271 in Haley, J. (Ed.), *Changing Families: A Family Therapy Reader*, New York, Grune & Stratton.

Rosen, J., *Direct Analysis*, New York, Grune and Stratton, 1953.

Rosenthal, A. (1970). Report on brief therapy research to the Clinical Symposium, Dept. of Psychiatry, Stanford University Medical Center, November 25.

Rosenthal, R. (1966). *Experimenter Effects in Behavioral Research*, New York, Appleton-Century-Crofts.

Saizman, L. (1968). Reply to the Critics, *American Journal of Psychiatry*, 6: 47-78.

Spiegel, H. (1967). Is Symptom Removal Dangerous? *Am. Journal of Psychiatry*, 123: 127-128.

Watzlawick, P., Beavin, J., & Jackson, D. (1967). *Pragmatics of Human Communication*, New York, W. W. Norton.

Watzlawick, P., Weakland, J., Fisch, R. (1974). *Change: Principles of Problem Formation & Problem Resolution*, New York, W. W. Norton.

Wender, H. (1968). The Role of Deviation-Amplifying Feedback in the Origin and Perpetuation of Behavior, *Psychiatry*, 31: 317-24.

# CHAPTER 5

# Communication Theory and Clinical Change[1]

## *John H. Weakland*

### I. "The reader is warned"— John Dickson Carr

Titles, like other labels, are often best met with critical wariness, including this one. "Communication Theory and Clinical Change" is accurately descriptive, since I will indeed discuss both communication theory and clinical change —here taken as purposeful intervention into problems on an individual and family scale, although the view involved is also more broadly applicable to human behavior and change. The apparently insignificant little word *and,* however, is perhaps the most important and potentially troublesome part of the title. It indicates, but probably does not adequately caution, that I will here be fundamentally concerned with the relationship between theory and practice. Since family therapy is increasingly a field of *practice,* and theorists and practitioners are, ordinarily, two different and separate breeds, discussion focused on this relationship may seem labored and beside the main point to many family therapists. The matter may be made still worse by the fact that "Communication and Clinical Change" is a large subject to cover in a small

---

[1] Reprinted from *Family Therapy: Theory & Practice,* Philip Guerin, (Ed.)., New York: Gardner Press, Inc., 1978. *Note:* The views expressed in this article are the formulation and responsibility of the author individually. Nevertheless it is certain that they reflect long experience at Mental Research Institute and it is probable that most of the author's Institute colleagues would generally agree with them.

compass, requiring severe selection and condensation. Accordingly, detailed information and illustrative examples will be minimal here—though amply available elsewhere (Watzlawick, Beavin-Bavelas, & Jackson, 1967; Watzlawick, Weakland, & Fisch, 1974; Watzlawick & Weakland, 1977); rather, I will outline the ideas and relationships I see as most basic, because they are general—not in the sense of "vague," but of broad relevance.

My aim here, that is, is not to get down to cases, but to get down to basic ideas and how they relate to getting down to cases. But since very different conceptions of communication and family therapy co-exist today, what seems basic and clear to the author and some of his colleagues may seem to others interested in theory to be on the wrong track, or to oversimplify complex and serious matters.

In short, the communicative task proposed here, even if it is possible, may be rather fruitless. But let us get on with the attempt, and since the going will be difficult in any case, start with the relationship of theory and practice in general.

## II. Theory and Practice

*Theory* has various meanings. As used here, in a broad but particular way, theory refers to whatever general concepts and principles a person holds in connection with some area of knowledge and action—in essence, a view or mental model of some matter. A theory, in this sense, may be less explicit, comprehensive, and systematic than the scientific ideal; indeed, people may even claim their ideas and behavior are a-theoretical. Yet even in such cases, a general view or model, often quite systematic and consistent, can usually be readily inferred from a reasonable amount of observation of their behavior—that is, specific actions and related statements. And such a model is always important in understanding the area of behavior to which it relates. It outlines what is taken as important or not important, logical or illogical, to be pursued or to be avoided, even what is possible or impossible. That is, we do not think and act in direct relation to reality, but in relation to some theory, view, or model—the term chosen is not important—of reality. Accordingly, any theory held, whether it is explicit or implicit, simple or complex, neatly organized or a melange of bits and pieces, has important practical consequences. To take an obvious example, if a therapist believes pathology is located within an individual, he may prescribe drugs or do analytic work, but he will not practice family therapy; this would not "make sense." And despite common complaints about the illogicality of human behavior, it seems more generally the case that people, including therapists, do behave logically in terms of their own premises—often, when the premises are questionable, all too logically, whatever the outcome.

It is, of course, common knowledge that theory can and has obscured as well as clarified, has caused difficulty as well as been helpful. Many and varied examples of this exist in history generally and the history of science in particular. In our own field, the family therapy movement itself has in considerable part arisen out of criticism of theories of individual psychopathology and treatment.

It would appear, though, that theory is apt to promote difficulty or error in practice not because of its inherent nature—and in any case practice necessarily involves theory as defined here—but primarily under certain circumstances: 1) When theory is neglected—usually by being left largely implicit. Then it is more difficult to make any critical examination of the kind of premises held, or of their consistency, or any comparison of expectations with observable events. 2) When theory is exalted—taken not as a useful view and tool, but as "reality" or at least a close approach to this ideal goal. Then theory tends to become an ultimate standard according to which all else must be decided, done, and judged. 3) It is curious to note that these two apparent opposites are both likely to occur in relation to the same situation—the downgrading of the immediate data of observations and statements from primary to secondary importance, and a corresponding elevation of interpretation, as the means to some deeper and more profound knowledge. In the one case, this usually involves emphasis on the clinician's empathy or intuition; that is, special personal insight that is not open to being challenged. In the other, theory reached via elaborate constructs and chains of inference becomes so grand and complex that if any discrepant data appear, these often are easily explained away or incorporated by further theoretical elaboration of similar kind, rather than revising and simplifying the theory (Kuhn, 1962).

On the view of theory stated earlier, no theory can be complete or perfect. A theory by this definition is a simplification, a tool for use in facilitating understanding and action (including transmission of ideas and techniques to others), and therefore is to be judged only by the results of its use. Generally, however, it appears best to have one's theory made as explicit as possible, and as simple and as closely related to data of direct observations as the subject of interest permits. The basic ground for this preference is that the terms and implications of such a theory, and its results in use, can be most readily subjected to critical survey.

In the more specific situation where one is involved, as we all are, in acting in some field as a practitioner, the importance of considering the relationship between theory and practice only becomes intensified—since professional work specifically implies deliberate behavior and operational expertise based on some general understanding. And what this understanding is, the view held of the field, largely determines what actions will be taken, the results of these actions, and even their evaluation.

Our own field, for instance, might be most broadly defined as concerned with dealing professionally with human events and actions that—being seen as strange, deviant, or destructive—presenting problems either to others, or to the actor himself. The corresponding basic questions are: What is the nature of such situations? What is their cause? What should be done about them? Historically among laymen and professionals there have been two main lines of explanation for such difficult or puzzling human situations, both for individuals and for groups of persons seen collectively—general views, with variations on each theme. On the one hand, human events and especially problems have been seen as the consequence of powerful impersonal forces, external to the realm of human behavior. Such forces may be supernatural, physical, or even social in so broad a sense as to be not personal—fate, God's will or demons, climate or geography, the economic system. To this class of large and powerful forces, in our day might be added certain minute but powerful factors, such as microbes and drugs.

Alternatively, human problems have been seen as the consequence of inherent personal factors—physical, mental, or moral attributes characteristic of an individual, or of a group of individuals, that determine their bad or mad behavior. And in some instances, such as with climate and racial character, or genetic theories of behavior, these two broad lines of interpretation may overlap.

These broad theories have correspondingly broad implications and expectable consequences which often are similar despite the apparent polarity of the two views. On the *nature* of human problems, both are concretistic. That is, they lead to seeing problems in an external and isolated way, apart from the viewer and from the flow of his ordinary life, as separate phenomena, existing in themselves. Correspondingly, the nature of such a problem is apt to be seen as rather plain or self-evident. The important question is then not its *what,* but its *why.* As to *cause,* such isolated and external viewing of problems is naturally accompanied by simple linear cause—effect theories; at the extreme (but a common extreme), "What is *the* cause of this problem?" Also, the cause is predefined as external to the person or persons defining the problem. The cause is "out there" in the external world, or in someone else, except—which is which is hardly a real exception—when it is in me, but not of me: I am doing something, but only involuntarily. Finally, there are corresponding implications about the *handling* of problems. To the idea of a single ultimate cause, there corresponds a search for overall or final solutions. The impersonal forces view leads either toward resigned acceptance—"Nothing can be done"—or to a call on some other external and higher power—God, a leader or science—for a major countereffort. The "someone is bad or mad" view may also lead to helpless pessimism, but it is more apt to lead to some combination of blame plus attempts, either hostile or supposedly benevolent, to change that other someone or ones, usually in a major way.

Of course there are human difficulties for which one of these views may be most appropriate, such as the kinds of concrete and practical difficulties immediately consequent on storm or earthquake, economic depression, accident, or sudden physical illness. But the problems people typically bring to psychotherapists are not like these. Clinical problems may arise out of such concrete difficulties, although more often no striking or dramatic origin is apparent; but in either case what is characteristic is helplessness, manifested either by inaction or confused activity, in the face of persisting difficulties that are escalating or have reached an impasse.

Here a model of problems based on the idea of communication and interaction may be more appropriate. Certainly such a model is fundamentally different in focus and implications from both of the views outlined above. From such a view, problems are seen as primarily involving ongoing behavior and interaction between persons in some system of social relationships. The relevant questions concern *what* is going on, which is not taken as self-evident; *how* does this continue when people want things to be different; and *how* can the functioning of the system be altered for the better, though no solution will be final or perfect? All this is abstract and general, but has profound human implications. Problems are not conceived as separate, but on a human scale related to everyday behavior, and as interactive, a matter of joint responsibility: "All in it together" rather than "sick versus well" or "bad versus good" or "wrong versus right." While this spreads the burden of dealing with problems, it also implies a spreading of any gains. A joint enterprise has potential mutual benefits, rather than winners versus losers.

But this is only a broad outline of a view, a conception to be tested by its usefulness. In order even to approach such critical appraisal, it is necessary next to pursue matters much further—to indicate, at the least, how this view developed, to spell out its terms in more detail, and to state more specifically what such a view leads to in practice.

## III. Communication Theory—Development and Delineation

Even the very general communicative view just sketched, let alone the specifics to be added shortly, did not spring into being full blown, like Venus from the sea-foam. Rather, the view being presented here represents a distillate of a long developmental process involving a variety of interrelated observations and ideas. A brief account of this development may be useful in two ways. For a more extensive account, from a somewhat different viewpoint, see (5).

In the first place, a view of the circumstances out of which this view of communication and interaction arose may help clarify and delimit what we are talking about more concretely than formal definition alone can. Communication has become a catchword and a catch-all. It means one thing to people interested in the mass media. It means another to communications engineers, who are largely concerned with clear and economical transmission of rather simple messages. And it means a variety of different, usually ideal, things to patients who complain about "poor communication" as a family problem—or even to various family therapists hoping to promote "good" communication. All these are different from our primary concern with the nature of observable face-to-face communication, verbal and nonverbal, among members of a family or other ongoing social group, and its significance for the shaping of actual behavior.

In the second place, a developmental account gives further perspective on the relation of practice and theory by presenting a concrete example of how the interaction of a few basic ideas and a variety of exploratory observations led to the present view of communication, problems, and their handling, which is quite different from the view of problems and therapy held originally, and may be expected to alter further in the future. This developmental summary may appear somewhat disorderly. In this also it reflects an actual relationship between theory and practice, rather than the fitting of events to a myth. In a view common among scientists as well as laymen, science develops according to an orderly scheme, involving the formulating of hypotheses based on existing knowledge, testing these out empirically, affirming or altering the hypothesis in line with the results, and repeating the process. This may be so somewhere. It is not how communication theory and family therapy grew up in close relationship, at least in Palo Alto, to which this account mainly refers. One thing did lead to another, but not in so orderly and planned a way. Certainly at times, theory—a systematized view—was distilled from practice *post facto,* rather than leading to it, although the converse did occur at other times, if often not altogether clearly and deliberately.

The beginning of this present view of communication and interaction may be referred—as always, somewhat arbitrarily—to Gregory Bateson's research project on communication. This began in late 1952, and involved Jay Haley, John Weakland, William F. Fry, Jr., and later Don D. Jackson. Initially, there was nothing specifically clinical about this research, though it was housed in the Palo Alto VA Hospital. Rather, it was broadly concerned with communication in general, and especially with communicational paradoxes. For example, Epimenides the Cretan says, "All Cretans are liars." If he is telling the truth, he must be a liar, and vice versa. Drawing on the idea of Logical Types, which Whitehead and Russell had developed and used in *Principia Mathematica* to explain certain contradictions in mathematics, such paradoxes were seen as related to the existence of multiple levels of abstraction in language. This simple but basic idea was kept in mind while examining a wide variety of actual communication, ranging from the conversation between a ventriloquist and his dummy to the play of otters observed in the zoo. The otter studies led to the conclusion that even animals must be able to give classificatory or framing messages equivalent to "What I am doing is play," and this led from the original idea of multiple levels of abstraction to the view that, in human communication especially, there is no such thing as a simple message. Instead, people are always sending and receiving a multiplicity of messages, by both verbal and nonverbal channels, and these messages necessarily modify or qualify one another.

That is, not only must all messages be interpreted, but the significance of any message singled out for attention cannot be determined from that message alone. It always depends also on how it is qualified—modified, reinforced, contradicted, specially framed ("When you call me that, *smile!*"), or whatever—by other simultaneous, preceding, or following messages. These (along with the setting, the relationship between the communicating parties, and so on) form part of the *context* which must be considered in interpreting any such message.

Moreover, the significance of a message is not just a matter of meaning, in the sense of information, but of behavioral influence. There is some message that indicates whether it is a serious bite or a playful nip, but this also largely determines whether more play or a fight will be the response. It is, of course, no discovery to note that messages can affect behavior; this is only common knowledge. It is an important further step, however, to insist that rather than *some* messages being informative and some directive, *all* messages have the two aspects labeled in the earlier work of Ruesch and Bateson (1951) as report and command. This key idea has been elaborated and discussed in other terms as well, including the expressive and effective aspects of messages, information and influence, and content and process in communication. Regardless of the specific terminology, this served to focus attention on the pervasiveness of communicational influence, which may be most important to note and understand precisely when it is complex, subtle, indirect or covert, rather than obvious. Another important idea was the recognition that unlike physical influence, in which a passive object is moved by and in proportion to the magnitude of an external force, communicational influence operates by activating and directing the energy of the receiver of a message. Therefore, small signals may easily have large effects, and still further multiplication of effect can occur when one signal frames the interpretation of many others, as often occurs. For these two reasons, then, the potential importance of communicational influence on behavior is great, and should never be neglected.

The project next took its first step from concern with communication in general toward involvement with clinical matters, by beginning to examine the communication of schizophrenics, being surrounded by this fascinating material in our VA Hospital setting. Schizophrenic speech (like their "crazy" behavior) was then generally thought to be incomprehensible nonsense. But the matter began to look quite different when actual samples were tape-recorded for repeated study and examined in context, with attention not just on the schizophrenic's words in isolation, but also on those of the interviewer, and the institutional environment as well. A new view was also promoted by having in mind our prior insight that most communication does not consist of simple declarative statements (an ideal of normality to which schizophrenic talk ordinarily was implicitly compared), but of a complex of mutually qualifying messages, including some which indicate how others should be interpreted—again, whether as a serious bite or a playful nip. This, too, is not really a new idea. Everyone knows that there are humorous, ironic, sarcastic, playful, and other kinds of messages as well as simple factual statements. But this knowledge had not been applied to schizophrenic communication, presumably because this, defined as "crazy," was viewed as separate and different in kind. Once we began to examine it in the same way as other communication, using the same general ideas, it appeared that if regarded as metaphoric in style—only lacking in the usual signs of metaphor, such as "It's like ..." or the use of conventional, familiar metaphors—much schizophrenic speech, otherwise unintelligible, made comprehensible sense. Even this lack of clear interpretative signs might be explained by considering that hospitalized patients could well be cautious and defensive, like members of the underworld relying on their private argot.

These notions received further support when we found that if we responded to patients' statements as metaphorical—instead of the common response of taking them literally, and trying to get the patient to acknowledge their illogic or unreality, a covert form of arguing with the patient—they then spoke more plainly. Different communication led to different communication. Somewhere along the line we began to see, perhaps aided by our prior insight that report and command are matters of analytic distinction rather than separate kinds of messages, that communication and behavior are not separate and different, but essentially the same thing viewed from different perspectives. Communication occurs only through the observation and interpretation of behavior, while all behavior in the presence of another is potentially communicative. (As a special case, one person can be both sender and receiver.) Which aspect is emphasized or seen as primary is only a matter of the point of view and purpose of the observer at a given moment.

In short, one thing had led to another until at this stage the research was already pursuing the study of the relationship of communication and behavior into the realm of "pathological" communication and behavior. But it was doing so on the basis of the same ideas about the complexity of communication, and its related ubiquitous, powerful, and complex behavioral influence as before, and with similar methods of close observation and study. That is, we were conceptually treating the abnormal the same as the normal, and moving progressively toward explaining things positively by inclusion—how does schizophrenic speech make sense in relation to speech in general—rather than negatively and by exclusion—how is it "illogical." Although this is a basic principle in scientific explanation, the principle is often breached in dealing with the abnormal, which is set apart, beyond the pale. In avoiding this, we were helped by the anthropological background of some of the research team. Anthropologists have traditionally been involved in the task of making sense out of apparently strange or bizarre behavior by viewing it in relation to other behavior, building up a view of a patterned whole within which each item has an understandable place and function. In any event, although many of our basic ideas were not novel, we were now involved in pursuing them toward wider limits: Just how much and what kinds of behavior (in the widest sense, including speech, actions, feelings, even bodily functioning) might be understood and accounted for on a basis of communicational influence, before having recourse to other avenues of explanation such as instincts or other genetic factors, biochemistry, early childhood events, or whatever? This line of inquiry, in fact, is still far from exhausted.

With our new view of the nature of schizophrenic communication, we next approached the question, "How is it that patients communicate in this fashion?" One part of our answer to this is implicit in what was said about the hospital context—quite possibly, such speech serves a defensive or protective function. Our other concern was with how schizophrenics might *learn* to communicate in such a way—essentially, "To what pattern of communication would such speech be an appropriate response, in some sense?" This also arose naturally out of our anthropological background, since by training and experience anthropologists commonly look for how behavior is learned in structured contexts of social interaction.

This inquiry about learning was pursued in part speculatively, by applying general knowledge about learning principles and multiple levels of messages to our characterization of schizophrenic speech; and in part by further empirical study. Since we had no way to reliably observe the past communicative background of our subjects, we started with what was directly observable, the communication of currently schizophrenic patients with their family members, especially young adult patients and their parents. Again this involved tape-recording and repeated close study. Out of such work came the concept of the "double-bind" (Bateson, Jackson, Haley, & Weakland, 1956), which described schizophrenic speech and other symptomatic behavior as a response to incongruent messages of different levels, within an important relationship, and where both escape from the field and comment on the incongruity were blocked. In the present context, the details of this formulation are less important than its general nature (Weakland, 1974), which is an attempt to produce a communicational explanation of crazy behavior by relating it to an identifiable pattern of communication within the family system from a functional view—that is, how the patient's behavior fits in and makes a certain kind of sense within a certain peculiar but observable communicational context.

In fact, things seemed to fit together so well in the here and now that we felt little need to move back toward the preschizophrenic days of the patient and family. Rather, our focus on the present system increased as we studied the interaction of schizophrenics and their families. Up to this stage, we had mainly studied dyadic interaction. Even in this, it had soon become evident that ordinary distinctions between "sender" and "receiver," or stimulus" and "response" were also analytic artifacts, essentially a matter of imposing punctuation on an ongoing system of communicative interaction. Since we describe and explain mainly by means of language, which involves discrete units and linear structure, such punctuation may be analytically useful or necessary. Certainly, it is important to recognize that the participants in any system of interaction regularly impose similar punctuation (which could also be seen as a larger scale example, applied to sequences, of that interpretation which is always involved in communication), and in ways that can be of major practical importance. For instance, many clinical problems involve punctuation directly paralleling that very commonly seen in children's quarreling: "You started it!" ("I'm only reacting to what you did.") "No, you started it first!" From a broader viewpoint, however, such punctuation, as well as being a source of conflict, is inaccurate and inappropriate. There is no "starting point" in an ongoing stream of interaction; the simple linear model of cause and effect is not appropriate. When we began to examine the more complex, yet highly patterned and repetitive interaction occurring in families, it became even clearer that the relevant epistemological model is one derived not from mechanics, but from cybernetics, where the focus is on the structure of interaction within some ongoing system.

Rather than pursuing our family studies into the preschizophrenic past, then, if this were possible, we concentrated on present functioning, and rapidly also became involved in looking toward the future. That is, motivated both by positive hopes, and by feeling the danger of being engulfed into their system while interviewing such families, we began attempts to change the going system in schizophrenic families for the better. These attempts were also promoted by observations that hospitalized patients who improved with individual treatment and were sent home often soon reappeared for further hospitalization, as well as by some early experience of Dr. Jackson with various members of patients' families.

This, then, was the beginning of family therapy in Palo Alto based on a communicational view of behavior (Jackson & Weakland, 1961). (At about the same time, of course, various others were also beginning to work with families from a variety of backgrounds in experience and viewpoint.) While neither our ideas nor our related techniques were fully and clearly formulated at this point, they appeared promising. And it was only a modest and natural next step—especially since schizophrenia was both a most difficult problem and one whose varied manifestations seemed to include much that was also characteristic of other kinds of clinical problems—to explore the relevance and use of family therapy as a general treatment approach. Where this has led, in terms of clinical practice and related theory, can now be described.

## IV. Problems, Persistence, and Change

The communicational view of behavior and related ways of dealing with problems developed gradually, with one thing leading to another, and action at times preceding formulation. In addition, some ideas—and certainly many specific terms—that were important or necessary as part of this development in retrospect no longer have the same importance. Put bluntly, a sizable part of our work on communication now appears related to digging ourselves out of individual-centered, depth-psychological views of behavior, problems, and therapy in which we originally were imbedded, rather than to any elaborate creation of new views. Once perceived, the ideas about communication and behavior basic to a communicational approach to treatment appear as rather few and rather simple, if not obvious. This, of course, is not to say there are no difficulties involved in sticking to these ideas in areas where one has learned well to understand matters in another way, or in applying them in specific, often apparently chaotic or confusing situations.

The two central ideas—of equal importance and closely interrelated—from which all else logically flows are: 1) that specific behavior of all kinds is primarily an outcome or function of communicative interaction within a social system; and 2) that "problems" consist of persisting undesired behavior.

On this view, unless there exists clear and clearly relevant evidence—not just a possibility, or ambiguous signs of some other significant causal factor such as organic pathology, observed behavior should be considered as structured and maintained primarily by current communicative interaction within some ongoing system of social relationships. This means *all* behavior, good or bad, voluntary or involuntary, normal or pathological. Indeed, if anything, this view should be applied most deliberately to unusual or abnormal behavior, for it is behavior labeled as such that most needs explanation—as a therapist once told an inquisitive patient, "Neither you nor I need to explain what is normal"—and that is most apt to be explained by different and special means. The relevant system of interaction is usually the family, but other systems such as school or work organizations may be important in some cases.

Clearly, this view puts an emphasis on observable communication—statements and actions—in the here and now. Similarly, the kinds of problems that people bring to therapists are seen as matters of currently persisting (or worsening) difficult, deviant, or symptomatic behavior. (Transient behavior may be unpleasant, but nothing need be done about it; by definition, it will pass.) Two closely related but distinguishable elements are involved in this: the more or less objectively observable behavior, and how it is judged and labeled by the patient or others associated with him. This distinction is important because in some cases—for instance, parents' over-anxious concern about ordinary childish mischief—the judgment, more than the behavior it labels, makes the problem. In either case, though, we see the problem as one of interpersonal behavior—what is being done, or how something is being labeled—neither as something more internal and personal, nor more external and impersonal.

This view of the nature of behavior and problems has several immediate and profound implications for treatment. First, the question, "What is wrong with this particular patient?" is largely irrelevant. This question is based on an individualistic view of problems, while from a communicational viewpoint the relevant question is, "What is going on in the system of interaction that produces the behavior seen as a problem?" or "How does this behavior fit in?"

Second, the concern common in many treatment approaches, "What is the *underlying* problem?" also is not relevant. If behavior is seen as primary, this "tip of the iceberg" idea no longer makes sense. Rather, the behavior complained of (or perhaps, as mentioned, its labeling as something requiring change) is the primary focus of treatment. This is not to say that other related behaviors may not need attention from the therapist. In fact, the communicational view clearly implies that the problem behavior must be considered in relation to other behavior. Nor does it mean that feelings, or past traumatic experience, for example, are simply to be neglected. It does mean that such factors are to be considered in relation to present behavior, not as somehow deeper or more fundamental, and are to be dealt with by appropriate changes in present behavior.

Somewhat similarly, the search for a root or original cause of any problem is foreign to the communicational view. This presumes a linear view of causality: A causes B, which then causes C. Such a view also subtly influences one to seek a cause corresponding in magnitude to the eventual problem. For instance: Schizophrenia is a dread syndrome, so somewhere behind it there must be great trauma, genetic deficiencies, biochemical abnormality—something big. But the picture is quite different on a cybernetic epistemology, which a view based on communication and interaction directly implies, and which indeed constitutes the most basic and general difference between interactional and individualistic approaches. From a cybernetic view, attention is focused on the structure of the system of interaction, and especially on its feedback loops. And where there is positive feedback—more of A leads to more of B, which leads to more of A, and so on—large effects can readily arise from minimal initial events. In more ordinary terminology, problems arise by snowballing, or vicious circles (Maruyama, 1963; Wender, 1968). Similarly, though this has received less consideration and investigation, the cybernetic epistemological view also raises the possibility that there may be no necessary or close relationship between the origin of a problem and its particular nature as ordinarily conceived—that is, the "diagnosis." For both size and shape of problems, any original precipitating event or difficulty may be of minor importance, and how it was dealt with in the environing system the main thing.

From this point of view, for the full blown problems that reach therapists' offices, the central question is not one of origins, but one of organization and persistence: "What behaviors in the ongoing system of interaction are functioning, and how, to maintain the behavior seen as constituting the problem?" This also fits with the idea that problems consist of behavior; that is, a problem is not something that simply exists in itself, a passive concrete object, but something that exists only in continuous or repeated performance. Furthermore, such a view centers on matters open to current inquiry, with a minimum of inference about unobservable past or intrapsychic events. For example, if a person says "isolation" is a problem, it is highly pertinent to consider how he behaves to avoid other people and to keep them from making contact with him, and to inquire, of course judiciously, about this.

Finally, at this general level, the resolution of problems correspondingly appears as primarily requiring a change of the problem-maintaining behaviors so as to interrupt the vicious positive feedback circles, and the therapist's main task as promoting such changes. Such alternative behaviors are always potentially open to the patient and other members of the system, but ordinarily it is not possible for them to change their usual but unsuccessful problem-solving behaviors on their own; those who can, do so, and therefore do not reach our offices. The therapist's job, accordingly, is to find and apply means of intervention that will help them make such changes, and the test of both specific interventions and the general approach is highly pragmatic: Do beneficial changes occur?

This outlined interactional approach to problems and treatment is clearly different from that of individual psychodynamic therapy, but the principles stated are still broad and general. A number of rather different views of family interaction and techniques of family therapy, involving different explicit or implicit emphases on structure, on good versus bad communication, on process versus content, and so on could largely fit with these principles. Discussion of such variants would be too lengthy here, and perhaps confusing. Instead, only the particular approach developed by MRI's Brief Therapy Center will be specifically described. The members of the Center see this particular approach as exemplifying a further refinement, boiling-down, and direct application of the most essential principles of the communicational view—though others, of course, may see it as a departure from the classic mold of family therapy.

Two further specifications of views already stated are important in the Center's approach and practice. First, while the origin of problems is not a vital question on the communicational view, one important aspect of the genesis of problems seems related to the crucial question of problem maintenance. In our experience, it appears that the problems brought to therapists commonly arise from difficulties of everyday life that have been mishandled by the parties concerned. Although such difficulties may at times involve special or unusual events—accidents, sudden illness, unexpected job loss—most commonly they involve adaptation to an ordinary life change or transition, such as marriage, childbirth, entering school, and so on. The mishandling involved may range from ignoring or denying difficulties on which action should be taken, to attempts to actively resolve difficulties that need not or cannot be resolved, with a wide area between where action is needed but the wrong kind is taken. Bad handling certainly does not correct, and usually increases, the original difficulty, which is then apt to be relabeled as a "problem," which is usually met by more of the same or similar inappropriate handling, leading to exacerbation or spread of the difficulty —and so on and on. That is, instead of viewing the cause and the nature of any problem as separate and different, we see the same essential process involved in problem formation as in problem maintenance. Rather similarly, we do not sharply separate chronic from acute problems, but see chronic ones as merely involving mishandling for a longer time. In short, the central focus of this view is not on difficulties as such—life is full of these, even for the most normal—but on their handling, for better or for worse.

Second, though quite consonant with the first point, our clinical observations indicate that usually it is precisely the ways people are trying to handle or resolve their problems that constitute or include those behaviors which are maintaining the problem in question. This of course is unrecognized by the participants in a problem situation. While we recognize that there are some payoffs from any system of interaction, even one full of problems, we do not see these as central in problem maintenance, nor as any major obstacle to change. The situation is not that bad—though in a way it is worse. Rather, our view is that people generally are well-intentioned and trying to improve things as best they know how; but what they see as the right and logical thing to do in the circumstances—often the *only* right thing and often supported by prevailing cultural views—is not working. The therapist's job, then, is apt to be the unenviable task of getting people to change that which they are apt to be clinging to most strongly. Correspondingly, to produce beneficial results, the therapist may have to promote remedies that might appear quite illogical to those most immediately concerned, and perhaps to many others as well.

Our overall treatment plan and procedures follow directly from these basic principles. Since our treatment focus is symptomatic, in a broad sense, we want first to get a clear statement of the presenting complaint, in terms of the specific, concrete behavior involved, and how this constitutes a problem. We attempt to get this information primarily by simple means such as direct questions, requests for clarification and examples, and asking for order of importance if a number of complaints are mentioned. Where more than one person is present, we ask each to state the main problem as he sees it, assuming their views may differ.

Next, we ask in a similar concrete way what the patient and any involved others are doing to try to handle the problem, based on our view that problems only persist if somehow maintained by other behavior, and that the locus of this ordinarily lies in peoples' efforts to deal with or resolve the problem. In our experience, when specific information on problem handling is obtained, and is considered in this light, problem-maintaining behavior often appears rather evident. For instance, it does not take any special skill, but just some objectivity and perspective, to see that the person with a sexual problem who works at performance is likely to make things worse rather than better by seeking to do the spontaneous voluntarily; or that the parents who tell a truant child what a wonderful experience and opportunity school offers are producing alienation rather than compliance. In some cases, of course, problem-maintaining reinforcements may be more difficult to perceive. They may be more complex or subtle; they may involve contradictory messages by the same or different persons; or the therapist's own accepted views about sensible behavior may obscure his observation of actual interaction and its effects.

Third, we ask all parties involved to state their minimal goal of treatment—that is, what observable behavioral change, at the least, would signify some success in the therapy. This is a difficult question for most patients to answer concretely, but an important one. Just to pose it conveys that change is possible, that it should be judged by observable behavior, and that small changes can be significant. According to our cybernetic view, if a small but significant change can be made in what appeared a major and hopeless problem, this is likely to initiate a beneficent circle and lead on to more progress. In contrast, pursuing vague or global goals is apt to lead only to uncertainty and frustration.

In addition to these three specific questions, two other matters are important from the outset, although information on these is gained more from close attention than direct inquiry. It is important to decide who is the main client—the "customer" for treatment. This means the person who most wants to see real change in the problem situation, usually because he or she is most concerned or hurting from it. This need not be the identified patient, or the person who makes the initial contact with the therapist. A wife may call to arrange an appointment for a drinking husband, or parents bring in a child who is failing in school. In such cases, unless the identified patient clearly indicates he personally is seriously concerned about the behavior in question, which often is not the case, we would if possible arrange to work primarily with the complainant—the wife or the parents. If one takes the idea of interaction in systems seriously, it follows that effective intervention can be made through any member of the system. Family therapy in this view does not consist of having everyone present in the therapist's office (although this may at times be desirable for information gathering or strategic purposes), but in working from an interactional *viewpoint.* And usually intervention can be most effectively made with the chief complainant, the person concerned enough to do something different.

For a similar reason, we attempt as soon as possible to grasp each client's "language"—the ideas and values that appear central to him. If people are to be moved to change their behavior, especially rapidly and in regard to behavior they believe is already logical and right, the therapist must perceive and utilize existing motivations and beliefs. Otherwise, his advice, however good, is likely to be ignored or opposed.

Once these inquiries and observations have been made, the therapist plans a related treatment strategy. That is, he concisely formulates the main presenting problem, and judges what behaviors are most central in maintaining it. He decides on a goal of treatment, estimating what concrete behavior would be the best sign of appropriate positive change. In all of this he of course takes full account of what the patients and others have said. But since on this view the therapist is an active and deliberate change agent someone being paid to exert influence expertly and beneficially—the responsibility for final decision is his. Even if his formulations agree with the patient's, it is the therapist who is deciding to proceed on this basis. Once the goal of treatment is determined, the therapist must consider intermediate steps, and the means to achieve them. What changes in the behavior of the patient, or others involved in the problem, are needed to approach the goal; and what interventions might be effective in promoting these changes?   In general, the therapist will aim to interdict the problem maintaining behaviors he perceives. The substitution of opposite behaviors for these will often be promoted, both to insure appropriate and adequate change, and because it is difficult for anyone just to stop doing something.

And since patients are already doing what they consider right, such changes can only rarely be accomplished by giving direct behavioral instructions on what to avoid or what to do. Instead, effective intervention usually requires reframing. That is, the problem situation must be redefined in such a way that the original motivations and beliefs of the persons involved now lead toward quite different behavior.

Beyond this, intervention rapidly becomes too particular a matter to be pursued further here. There is no "good intervention" as such; what is effective and useful always depends on the circumstances of the particular case. Of course this is true of every aspect of actual practice. One must get down to particulars, and often in difficult circumstances, with people who are confused, anxious, angry, or dogmatic. Even in the first and simplest matter of inquiring what the problem is, practical difficulties may arise, and special techniques or interventions may be needed just to get necessary basic information.

More has been said about the practice of change elsewhere (Watzlawick, et. al., 1974; Weakland, Fisch, Watzlawick, & Bodin, 1974), and despite its importance, this is not the main focus here. Rather, I have outlined a communicational view of behavior and problems, to show how certain general principles and procedures relate to this view—a framework for guiding and evaluating the more specific thought and action that practice necessarily involves.

## References

Watzlawick, P., Beavin-Bavelas, J., & Jackson, D. (1967). *Pragmatics of Human Communication.* New York: Norton.

Watzlawick, P., Weakland, J., & Fisch, R. (1974). *Change.* New York: Norton.

Watzlawick, P., & Weakland, J. (Eds.) (1977). *The Interactional View,* New York: Norton.

Kuhn, T. (1962). *The Structure of Scientific Revolutions.* Chicago: University of Chicago.

Haley, J. (1976). Development of a Theory: The Rise & Demise of a Research Project. In C. Sluzki & D. Ransom (Eds.), *Double Bind: The Foundation of the Communicational Approach to the Family,* New York: Grune & Stratton.

Ruesch, R., & Bateson, G. (1951). *Communication: The Social Matrix of Psychiatry.* New York: Norton, 1951.

Bateson, G., Jackson, D., Haley, J., & Weakland, J. (1956). Toward a Theory of Schizophrenia, *Behavioral Science*, 1, 251-64.

Weakland, J. (1974). The Double-Bind Theory' by Self-Reflexive Hindsight, *Family Process*, 13 (1974), 269-77.

Jackson, D., & Weakland, J. (1961). Conjoint Family Therapy: Some Considerations on Theory, Technique, and Results, *Psychiatry*, 24, 30-45.

Maruyama, M. (1963). The Second Cybernetics-Deviation Amplifying Mutual Causative Processes, *American Scientist*, 51(1963), 1~79.

Wender, P. (1968). Vicious & Virtuous Circles: The Role of Deviation Amplifying Feedback in the Origin & Perpetuation of Behavior, *Psychiatry*, 31, 309-24.

Weakland, J., Fisch, R., Watzlawick, P., & Bodin, A. (1974). Brief Therapy: Focused Problem Resolution, *Family Process*, 13, 141-68.

# CHAPTER 6

# The Strategic Approach

## John H. Weakland and Richard Fisch

### Abstract

*Weakland and his associates (Watzlawick, Weakland, & Fisch, 1974; Weakland, Fisch, Watzlawick, & Bodin, 1974) have developed a brief therapy procedure that focuses on present observable behavioral interaction and uses intervention to change the ongoing system. In this model the client's problem is viewed as a social phenomenon that reflects some dysfunction within the system of interaction and is best treated by effecting some change in that system. Treatment is limited to 10 sessions and a 3-month follow up.*

The general view of problems and treatment underlying this approach is based on assumptions that are different from those often held about hyperactivity. The most fundamental assumption is that all one can ever have in attempting to understand and deal with human problems is a *view,* that is, a conception, rather than "the truth." The particular view held by the therapist is of great importance, because of its very real consequences. The view taken largely determines not only what one attends to and how one organizes what is observed in examining a problem, but also how one acts to handle it and what will result. For example, if hyperactivity is conceived to be a physiological problem, physical means of treatment, usually drugs, will naturally be utilized. If hyperactivity is considered a psychological problem in the usual sense, namely something related to a person's mental structure or functioning, some form of exploratory individual psychotherapy naturally follows as treatment. Weakland et al.'s view of the nature of human problems, different from both of these, is interactional. Unless there is clearly evident and relevant organic pathology, they consider the kinds of problems people bring to psychotherapists or often to physicians, including hyperactivity, to be matters of difficult, deviant, or symptomatic behavior. The two elements involved here are: first, the observable behavior, and second, how it is labeled and judged by the patient or others involved with him. All behavior is viewed as being primarily maintained and structured by interaction between people, especially in the family system, but also in other systems, such as the school for children and work situations for adults. Within this view the question "What is wrong with a particular individual?" is largely irrelevant, as is the search for the root cause of the problem, which presumes a linear idea of causality that is not relevant to this approach: Problems are regarded primarily as outcomes of everyday difficulties, usually involving adaptation to an ordinary life change or transition, that have been mishandled by the parties involved. Such mishandling may range from ignoring or denying difficulties on which action should be taken to attempts to actively resolve difficulties that need not or cannot be resolved, with a wide area in between where action is needed but the wrong kind is taken. When such ordinary difficulties are handled badly, things tend to snowball: bad handling increases the difficulty, soon relabeled as a "problem," then is usually followed by more of the same inappropriate handling, leading to exacerbation or spread of the difficulty, so that originally minor or common life difficulties may readily lead on to serious symptomatology.

Accordingly, the central question in this approach is "What behaviors in the ongoing system of interaction are functioning to maintain the behavior seen as constituting the problem?" The resolution of problems is seen as primarily requiring a change of the problem-maintaining behaviors so that the destructive spiraling effect is interrupted. The general treatment procedure stems directly from these basic principles. First the therapist inquires about the main problem or presenting complaint and attempts to get a clear statement of this in terms of specific concrete behavior. Next he inquires about what the patient and others who are involved are doing to try to handle the problem, because these problem-handling efforts are most likely to comprise the behaviors central to maintaining the problem. Then those who are involved are asked to state their *minimum* goal for treatment, that is, what observable behavioral change would signify some success in the treatment. This important question is a difficult one for most patients, but change can be most easily effected if the goal is clearly stated and, while significant, is small. If a small but definite change is made in a major but seemingly hopeless problem, this is likely to initiate a beneficial circular effect and lead on to more progress, whereas pursuing vague or global goals is apt to lead only to uncertainty and frustration. From the outset, an attempt is made through attentive observation and listening to grasp each client's "language," the ideas and values that are central to him, because the therapist must perceive and make use of existing motivations and beliefs if he is to change behavior that the patient already considers is right and logical. When all these inquiries and observations have been made, the therapist plans a treatment strategy based on his own summarization of the problem. He concisely formulates the main presenting problem, identifies the behaviors that are central in maintaining it, decides on a goal of treatment, and estimates what concrete behavior would be the best sign of positive change. In general, the therapist will want to prevent the occurrence of the behaviors seen as crucial to maintaining the problem, and often does this by substituting opposite behaviors for them. This latter step is generally done by reframing or redefining the problem situation in such a way that the original motives and beliefs of the persons involved will now lead to very different behavior. The following case study (Weakland & Fisch, 1975) illustrates the brief therapy procedure with two boys who had been diagnosed as hyperactive and who had both been on medication for several years. The case also serves as an excellent example of the damage that can ensue when labels that parents do not understand are arbitrarily attached to children, and no adequate follow-up procedures are provided to determine how the parents react to the diagnostic information they are given.

The family was referred by the Juvenile Probation Department. The father and mother were both in their early forties, their sons, Roy and Dennis, were 13 and 11. The father was rather quiet although he followed all of the discussions with lively interest; the mother, a rather nervous, bird-like woman who came armed with copious notes on the boys' behaviors and histories, was much more active during sessions than her husband. The boys were rather well-mannered and listened attentively, at times indicating quiet amusement at their parents' tales of woe and mischief.

The mother immediately went into great detail about the boys' long history of behavioral problems. Dennis and Roy had consistently posed problems for their teachers, were inclined to be obstreperous in class, their attention lagged, and schoolwork was done shoddily or incompletely. By the time they reached the fourth and fifth grades the school psychologist had defined their behavior as "hyperactivity" and possible "minimal brain dysfunction," and had urged the parents to seek medical evaluation. A physician agreed that they were suffering from "hyperactivity," placed them both on Ritalin, and, in later years, prescribed Thorazine.

The medication made some improvement, but not enough to let matters rest there. Further psychological evaluation showed that both boys were also psychologically handicapped, having "poor impulse control." The parents, highly conscientious, conventional and unimaginative people who were impressed by all these determinations, regarded the boys as seriously disturbed and saw their sons' "lack of impulse control" as placing them constantly on the brink of explosive catastrophe. In addition to cooperating with medical and school regimens, they set about to exert *continuous* surveillance of the children, setting aside their own social and personal needs to implement this task, which resulted in considerable social isolation for them.

The precipitating event for Probation Department intervention occurred in mid-January when Dennis took the family car for a half-hour joy-ride. The parents alerted police who waited at the home for the boy's return. When he appeared unscathed, the policemen simply left. But the incident left the parents panicked; they regarded the taking of the car as "impulsive out-of-control behavior," and a situation that called for immediate and extreme measures. They took Dennis to the Juvenile Hall, demanded his immediate admission, and requested that he remain there.

When the family was referred to us it was mid-April and Dennis was still detained in the Juvenile Hall. The family was seen for 10 sessions, spaced weekly; the parents were present for all interviews, the boys for only the first four. From the start, both parents stressed the severity of the boys' disabilities, minutely detailing the history of their troubles, the need for medications, the failure of all previous measures to "control" them and the utter hopelessness of the situation. In keeping with our treatment view of "speaking the client's language," the therapist earnestly agreed with their pessimism. This had the desired effect of reassuring the parents that, at last, they had found someone who really understood the seriousness of their plight, and they relaxed enough to agree, by the end of the third session, to take Dennis home from Juvenile Hall. The therapist was careful to frame that step, not as any improvement in Dennis, but as a necessity to see how really bad he was when all special controls were removed. He explained that, since our treatment program was a brief one, we had to get to the heart of the matter right away. As a concomitant step, he asked the parents to discontinue both boys' medications for the week since the Thorazine would also obscure the "illness." He then turned to the boys and pointedly instructed them that in the ensuing week they were to "be themselves" and not worry about getting into trouble since they had just heard their parents told to expect the worst. As was hoped, the parents reported in the following session that the week went much better than they had expected - enough better to convince them that neither boy required medication. The parents subsequently discontinued the medication.

In the fifth session the parents were seen alone and the therapist took a slightly divergent tack: the father had mentioned a problem with Roy, who was inclined to be aggressively defiant and, during one confrontation, had knocked his father down. The father simply took it and felt that he had handled it rather badly, but was at a loss as to what to do about such situations. He raised all kinds of objections to using force himself, to which the therapist rejoindered by redefining force as "therapeutic," stating, "If I were a son and felt my father couldn't protect himself, even against me, I would be fearful that he therefore couldn't protect me." This seemed to sit rather well with the father and the therapist added that such forceful action was well within the proper domain of an authority. Within the week, the father successfully put to use this new "therapeutic" permission with Roy.

After the sixth session, the therapist assessed the situation. Dennis was now back home, both boys were off medication and the parents were more relaxed. However, it was obvious that their feeling of control within the home was tenuous and the therapist felt that some additional step was needed to solidify their confidence. He probed for some everyday situation that, while in itself no major problem, signified to them their lack of control over the boys. The parents described such a situation. Either boy might be sent on some errand and instead of returning right away would "wander off." That these "wanderings off" were harmless meant little because to the parents it was a clear sign of a "lack of impulse control." Because they viewed it this way, the parents, on sending the boys on an errand, would give them overly detailed instructions regarding the errand, conveying great anxiety about "wandering off." Their very attempts to prevent the "wandering" were actually invitations to do so.

In the seventh session the mother suddenly announced, "This week there isn't anything I wouldn't trust Dennis with. I know he is in perfect control." When asked to explain this puzzling certitude, she said that she relied on her intuition. The therapist regarded her "intuition" as a serious obstacle to treatment that, if allowed to persist, could sabotage gains by bringing about a self-fulfilling prophecy. He suggested that such power to intuit could be converted into a sort of "sending set" to *project* thoughts, not only pick up another's thoughts. She was intrigued and expressed some interest in seeing what she could do about it. The therapist suggested that she attempt such an exercise when sending either of the boys on an errand, but it was emphasized that she would need to give the boys the most *minimal* instructions, otherwise, should they carry out the task successfully, she would have no way of knowing whether it was her fully detailed instructions or the new-found use of her "intuition." In the following session, the eighth, the mother reported two successful trials. In one instance, she had received a call from the school that Dennis was hanging around the bike racks and had failed to heed the bell signaling a new class. She then concentrated her thinking on him saying in her mind that he was to go right back into class, and a few minutes later received a call from school that Dennis had just returned to class. (This also illustrated the elaborate surveillance system the parents had set up, getting the school to call her at the slightest transgressions of the boys.) The other opportunity consisted of sending Roy on an errand and this trial went equally well. She acknowledged that this could be coincidence and the therapist agreed.

Termination of treatment was anticipated in the ninth session when they indicated quite clearly a higher level of confidence in their ability to control the children and expressed satisfaction with the boys both at home and at school. Treatment was terminated in the tenth session and in a follow-up evaluation three months later the parents reported that they were having no difficulties. The mother had tried using her "intuition" a couple of times after terminating treatment but had not done so since because they could trust the boys. More significantly, the parents reported they were finally resuming their social lives—going to a movie without the boys, inviting friends into the home and accepting invitations.

In summarizing this case, we might say that the "problem" was not the boys' misbehaviors but the attempted solution, chief of which was to originally define their misbehavior as "hyperactivity," "minimal brain dysfunction," and "lacking impulse control." This "solution" set the course for further medical, school, and parental "solutions" which produced an escalating and elaborate structure of anxious mishandling.

Procedures such as the therapist's use of the mother's belief in her intuitive powers have been criticized as "manipulative" and "deceitful." It is our opinion that the main criterion for the use of a therapeutic technique in medicine or psychiatry should be the immediate and/or long-term well-being of the patient. With this criterion it is also the therapist's responsibility to treat aftereffects of such a treatment procedure. In the case cited here it is unlikely that directing the mother to stop belaboring her sons with instructions would have been as effective as the approach chosen. The procedure described here was successful in terminating this tendency, the mother did not continue to rely on her intuition, and the therapist checked on this point at the 3-month follow up. It is interesting that critics of this general approach seldom question the clinical and experimental use of procedures such as placebos.

Before, we saw treatment as requiring the cessation of these "solutions." The parents were indicating the enormity of the burden required to maintain the view that the boys' difficulties were those of "hyperactivity," "minimal brain dysfunction," or "lack of impulse control." But they were overwhelmed and confused as to how to back off from that limb. It necessitated using their own "language"—concepts that were logical to them—but in a way that could allow them to redirect their efforts and bring about the putting to rest of a nonexistent "disease" and treat the boys as normal, albeit obstreperous, children.

## References

Watzlawick, P., Weakland., J., & Fisch, R. (1974). *Change—Principles of Problem Formation and Problem Resolution*, New York: W. W. Norton & Co.

Weakland, J., Fisch, R., Watzlawick, P., & Bodin, A. (1974). Brief Therapy: Focused Problem Resolution, *Family Process*, 13 (1), 141-168.

# CHAPTER 7

# "Family Somatics"
# A Neglected Edge[1]

### *John H. Weakland*

If I appear to sound a negative note in my title with "A Neglected Edge," it is because I take our conference theme, "The Growing Edge," seriously. The positive aim of growth can at times be served by negative—or at least critical—means. To cite an example especially relevant here, constructive criticism of individual treatment was a significant factor in Nate Ackerman's laying of foundations for family therapy. So I will make some critical comments in this paper about what we are not doing in one particular area, with the positive aim of stimulating useful thought and action.

Our field of interest, as stated on our journal's masthead, is "family study, research and treatment." There are ample grounds in our work, I believe, for an even wider definition: that we are concerned with applying an interactional systems viewpoint, focused mainly but not exclusively on family systems, to the study and better handling of human problems. Either statement, however, leaves undefined exactly what sort of problems are to be examined and treated. This seems all to the good, especially since ours is still a new field. It avoids premature closure, and the accompanying danger of possibly excluding potentially relevant problem areas from our purview—at least by formal definition.

[1] Originally published in P. Watzlawick & J. Weakland (Eds.), (1977) , *The Interactional View*, New York: W. W. Norton & Co. p. 375-387.

Nevertheless, such exclusion could still take place, in practice and in effect, simply by concentration of our interest and effort on certain areas and neglecting other possibilities. This paper will suggest that this has indeed been the case concerning the potential relevance of family interaction for illness generally—that is, including even clearly organic pathology—and will suggest possible steps toward rectifying this apparent neglect. This area of inquiry I have termed "family somatics," by an obvious analogy to "psychosomatics."

## Background

I am, of course, not maintaining that there is *no* current interest in disease from a family interaction viewpoint. Neglect, and even exclusion, are relative terms; in this instance, relative in two respects. First, disease appears to be receiving less attention from workers in the family field than it did formerly, although meanwhile our field has grown considerably. Second, this approach to problems of disease appears to receive scant attention overall, in comparison to the time, money, and effort expended on genetic, physiological and biochemical research.

When family interaction studies and family therapy were just getting started—only fifteen to twenty years ago—all of our work involved moving, somewhat tentatively, into new territory. Even if the problems involved were old; perhaps *especially* when they were old and therefore "known"—applying a new viewpoint made it a new ball game, and a dubious one to many observers holding established views. Nate Ackerman's interest in the family originally appeared, in the New York analytic context, a wild idea. The case was similar for the early work on schizophrenia and the family, which constituted a point of entry into wider family concerns for many—including Wynn, Bowen, and Lidz, as well as my Palo Alto colleagues and myself. When this work began, schizophrenia certainly was not generally seen, either by laymen or professionals, as a problem of interaction, especially current interaction. Rather, it was viewed by some in a very "mentalistic" way, and by more (at least among professionals) in a physiological framework, though with varying emphases on genetics, neurology, and biochemistry. This latter kind of opinion, indeed, is still very strong. Nevertheless, such uphill work based on the family interaction viewpoint produced significant and lasting contributions to the understanding and treatment of schizophrenia—that is, in an area where this viewpoint had widely been considered to be irrelevant to the nature of the disease.

Interest then developed at MRI (which I use for exemplification because of familiarity) in looking at some other more or less clearly "physical" problems—from asthma and ulcerative colitis at the more evidently psychosomatic end of the scale to coronary disease at the other. But although some suggestive ideas and observations developed, none of this work ever was pursued beyond a stage of preliminary inquiry—in part because of the untimely death of Don Jackson, in part because of changes in research funding, and in part because greater involvement in treatment as such.

If a broader view is taken, the situation appears much the same. The content of *Family Process* probably offers the best single indicator of work in our field. The first five volumes included just two articles clearly concerned with the family and physical illness. Bursten's (1965) article on "Family Dynamics, the Sick Role, and Medical Hospitalization," though interesting, is largely limited to an interest in family exacerbation or emphasis of existing disease. Meissner's (1966) article on "Family Dynamics and Psychosomatic Processes" is an important survey of psychosomatic ideas about a wide range of diseases—including duodenal ulcer, ulcerative colitis, hypertension, hyperthyroidism, arthritis, tonsillitis, tuberculosis, diabetes, cancer and leukemia—together with pertinent suggestions about the advantages of a family rather than individual viewpoint in considering the "psychological" factors in disease: "The awareness has grown in recent years that human disease, in addition to a pathology, also has an ecology. The understanding of disease, then, must comprehend the pertinent aspects of that ecology if it is to be at all meaningful. The patient's emotional involvement in the family system constitutes a major aspect of that ecology which we can no longer afford to ignore." (Meissner, 1966, p. *157*). Yet this paper was only a beginning, as Meissner himself recognized, a tentative formulation which might serve as a heuristic basis for further much needed study". And it has not been followed up as he hoped. In the next five volumes of *Family Process,* there is no article directly concerned with this area. At most, Spark and Brody's (1970) "The Aged Are Family Members" has some implicit relevance for the problem of senility. If anything, in view of the growth of publications in the journal, this evidence suggests a decline in interest in problems of physical illness. But relevant articles are so scarce at best that it is probably most accurate to conclude that this adventurous and promising, though difficult, line of work never really got off the ground.

This examination, however, has not considered the established field of psychosomatic medicine sufficiently. Perhaps relevant work has been done, but published only in its journals? This, however, also does not seem to be the case. A brief survey of *Psychosomatic Medicine* and *Psychosomatics* is enough to see how completely they are still concerned with an individualistic, or at most a mother-child orientation, to psychological factors in disease. And this point is documented extensively, though unintentionally, by Grolnick's (1972) recent *Family Process* article, "A Family Perspective of Psychosomatic Factors in Illness; A Review of the Literature." Grolnick obviously searched diligently for examples of "Family Perspective" as his 129 references attest. Yet again, many of his references are concerned with essentially psychological or hypo-chondriacal problems, and many deal with only individuals or dyads; very few are really concerned with the relationship of interaction patterns and physical illness.

In sum, since the early days referred to above, the family interaction view-point has become more widespread and family therapy in particular has be-come much more established, accepted and widely practiced; variations in therapeutic approach and technique also continue to develop. But it does not seem that there has been a parallel growth in the range or variety of problems that the interactional viewpoint is applied to practically, or even theoretically. Rather, treatment and even thinking and observation, are largely concentrated on problems which-at least to those associated with the field-now appear as plainly and manifestly emotional or behavioral in nature; that is, on the tradi-tional, though now relabelled, area of "psychopathology." Nor, meanwhile, has our basic interactional viewpoint appeared to spread and influence those more immediately concerned with "psychological" factors in illness to any significant degree.

Obviously, I am here proposing that efforts might be made to alter this situation—that family therapists and researchers might themselves devote more attention to problems of physical illness, and that we might also promote wider understanding and utilization of our interactional viewpoint among those already concerned with illness—certainly those involved in psychoso-matic medicine, and perhaps in medicine more generally. On the other hand, promoting such change would not be an easy task, and since so little work along these lines has actually been done, proposals for such action and change cannot be supported by much direct evidence of relevance and utility. As with all original research, if we had the sort of information hoped for, the work would not be needed; it is rather a question of proceeding on the basis of rea-sonable expectations.

In the circumstances, therefore, I will attempt to support my proposals by presenting: 1. A discussion of the rationale for work on illness and interaction-the general grounds for believing this approach relevant; 2. Suggestions of how such work might at least be begun; and 3. Some consideration of the probable consequences-both difficulties and benefits of such work.

## Rationale

The fundamental basis for investigating interaction and illness actually is obvious. There exists the same general situation that historically has been the basis for important research in many other areas: We know just enough to rec-ognize that there is much we don't know that might be significant. Most simply, there is some evidence that interaction can and does influence bodily functioning. Therefore, it *may* be significant for some or even all those sorts of functioning or dysfunctioning—this distinction being one of semantics and point of view—that we term illness. Yet it is equally plain that we know little, generally or specifically, about either the extent of this potential significance or its limits. A clue concerning major problems is at hand, but—some possible reasons will be mentioned later—we have not got on with the inquiry needed to determine whether this clue is of great, or only minor, significance for those problems.

It is not necessary here to set forth the existing evidence for the influencing of bodily function by social interaction in any detail. All that is required as a reasonable basis for inquiry—especially in the circumstances of general neglect of this area of possible relationships—is an indication that such influence is possible rather than impossible. And, in fact, evidence for the influencing of bodily function by interaction abounds. One could even fairly say that this is a matter of everyday common knowledge, among both laymen and medical men. Only it is conceived and phrased differently. Thus it is a matter of everyday experience that emotions often affect such bodily functions as blood circulation and hormonal secretion obviously and markedly. Such effects have also been studied scientifically at least since the days of Cannon (1920), and continuing reports of such work appear in the psychosomatic journals currently. Considerable changes in bodily function also can be rather readily produced in hypnosis. The question of more lasting and profound bodily changes, such as are involved in disease, is a more difficult one, but again both lay and professional observers—from Dunbar (1954) to Selye (1956)—have been seriously concerned with the significance of experience for the gravest diseases. Perhaps the worldwide folk belief connecting disease and evil personal influence should be considered more seriously. At least, Cannon (1942) believed death by witchcraft to be a real and scientifically explainable possibility. All in all, it seems that Herman's (1955) statement is quite a moderate and reasonable one: "That emotional phenomena accompany or lead to physical phenomena is undisputed. It is also well known that factors in the psychological pattern or events in the life of the patient have great influence on the progress or amelioration of the disease state."

Most of the above points simultaneously to the significance of this area and—but only implicitly—to the fundamental problem involved. That is, these views of bodily influence and changes largely focus on the individual, in relation to "emotions," on the hypnotic "state," or general "stress"; they fail to note that emotions, hypnosis (Haley, 1958), and stress all depend greatly on communicative interaction, which can be observed and studied. This, as mentioned, may be only a difference of conception and phrasing—but our own work with families is based on just such a difference, and has shown how important this can be for theory, research, and practice.

Thus there is usually under other names, considerable and varied evidence that bodily function can be and is influenced by communicative interaction. At the same time, much is unknown about what patterns may be significant for long-term or continuing effects on such functioning, let alone the matter of possible structural changes, and probably still less for particular diseases. Again, this means only that a field of great possible importance is lying open and fallow. Perhaps such relationships do not exist, or cannot be discerned with our present scientific resources. But perhaps they can, and we only know by trying, by checking it out. At this point, there may not be a total absence of such inquiry, but certainly such inquiry is minimal in comparison to individual-centered psychosomatic studies, let alone the enormous expenditures of time and money routinely poured into biochemical and physiological studies of disease.

We may also consider several different ways in which interaction might be relevant to illness somewhat more specifically. If, proceeding chronologically or developmentally, we begin with the onset or etiology of illness, there are at least three general ways in which interactional situations or patterns might be significant. First, a certain sort of interaction, presumably continuing over some length of time, might itself constitute the sufficient conditions for the beginning of a certain disease. "Itself" in this instance would not mean in isolation, but in connection with otherwise healthy persons and generally obtaining environmental circumstances. Probably, if any such instance exists, the sort of interaction involved would have to be very special, though this is not equivalent to obvious or blatant. It is not easy even to imagine a possible example, but this logical possibility should not be ignored. Second, a certain sort of interaction might constitute a necessary but not sufficient condition for the onset of a certain disease. That is, while the development of a disease might definitely require the presence of some virus or other noxious agent, it could concurrently require some particular sort of interactive situation for the agent to be effective. Therefore, attention should be paid to both aspects; even if an agent is essential, it should not be seen as *the* cause of its associated disease. In this connection, one might think of those many diseases whose active agents are ubiquitous or at least occur widely, but which only certain individuals actually develop. Such selectivity at present often does not seem well accounted for by strictly medical factors such as general health: interaction might be significant for susceptibility. It is even conceivable, and worth considering, that even if there is little or no correlation between specific interaction patterns and specific diseases, there may be some broader correlation—that is, that some form or forms of interaction may increase susceptibility to illness generally, with the particular disease contracted being dependent on other factors. Finally, there might be diseases for which certain sorts of interaction, while not necessary, would contribute as sensitizing or predisposing influences.

Once an illness exists, interaction may be relevant to its course and outcome, for better or worse. Such an influence might be direct—that is, one form of interaction might interfere with the body's functions of resistance and healing, while another might facilitate these, as hypnotic suggestion appears to do in certain cases. Less directly, yet perhaps equally significantly, interactive factors might function to help or hamper the useful application of medical treatment for a given problem. To take a relatively simple example, the success of current therapies for cancer depends greatly on whether the disease is recognized and treated early or not. As Shands (1960) and others have noted, failure of recognition in many cases appears to involve active avoidance or denial, not just the overlooking of minor signs; certainly interaction might be important in this.

In another respect, however, the interactional viewpoint might lead towards some useful questioning of this usual distinction between etiology and course of disease, with the related major emphasis on etiology that is especially common in research and public health work. Our own work in family research and therapy—again the early work on schizophrenia is a clear example, followed by many others—has largely involved such a shift of viewpoint and emphasis concerning behavioral problems. From seeking for some original etiology and linear causation of problems, we have moved toward much greater concern with circular causality involving feedback loops, and the corresponding importance of reinforcements that keep a problem going, or worsening. Evidence collected from this perspective suggests that how a problem got started—which may involve rather ordinary or minor matters—is often less important than what causes the problem to persist and develop. It is quite possible that such an orientation might also be very relevant for a new look at physical illness: again, we simply cannot tell *a priori.*

## Approaching Such Research

While it is not possible to lay out a specific research program in advance because so little is yet known about this area, this level of ignorance itself suggests certain broad guidelines for productive study. That is, such study should initially be correspondingly exploratory and flexible, guided by general principles rather than rigid prescriptions. Since what is specifically significant about interaction in relation to illness is not known, but the very subject of inquiry, any attempt to predetermine just what must be viewed and the means of viewing is apt to be not only useless but self-defeating. In such an enterprise, fixed targets and instruments can only focus attention on things that are prominent, or that one assumes *must* be important—but it is more likely that if these matters were significant, important discoveries would have been made from them already. Meanwhile, wide-ranging but careful scanning of the terrain is obstructed.

This, again, is the sort of approach taken in our early studies of schizophrenics and their families. It led to discerning the double-bind interaction pattern which, though actually fairly simple and plain, previously went undetected amid many inquiries seeking factors dramatic or drastic enough to account for such a dread illness, and much psychological testing bound up by categories precise but not pertinent. What people know must be important is not always what really matters.

In the present case, a similar approach might mean beginning with some form of natural history study, utilizing direct observation of interaction related to illness, rather than collection of masses of discrete data by questionnaires, for instance. This might be begun by interviewing and observing at length a small sample of families with a member having a particular sort of illness, and simply looking for any discernable patterns of interaction they have in common—as a first step.

A few tentative suggestions may be offered on the general orientation of such family interviews, although too much specificity still appears a greater danger than looseness. Beyond the ordinary gathering of family demographic data, interviews might initially be focused on three matters. First, the family's conception of the disease, its nature and its history—which might include inquiry about any similar previous disease in the same or preceding generations. Second, in what concrete ways the disease is presently a problem, for the patient and for other family members, in daily life. Third, how are the patient and other family members attempting to handle these problems? Where feasible, this might include investigation of their responses to any suggestions that could be made as to possibly more useful ways of dealing with the disease, since reactions to potential change are often especially illuminating about family behavior. Hopefully, examination of the data gathered in this way might lead to the perception of regularities in how particular diseases are conceptualized—their perceived nature, causes, who or what is to blame –and handling—by avoidance, frantic activity, reassurance or whatever, which might provide leads for further inquiry.

It is plain that the simple approach suggested above starts from existing identified cases of illness. Therefore, it may not relate most directly to the question of interactional causes of the illness, and it also involves the perennial worry that observed interaction may be mainly a result of the illness. Two factors seem to outweigh these potential difficulties, however. First, as suggested earlier, our professional experience, together with the whole theory of cybernetics and systems of interaction, increasingly suggests that the old distinction, cause vs. course of problems, may not be so valid or significant as formerly believed; it may even be a misleading focus for thought and observation. Second, this appears to be the only feasible way to arrange direct study of interaction related to illness at the start, and this is the most likely source of fresh observations and ideas. Later, perhaps, leads gained in this way might be used to search for cases of potential illness to be followed over time.

Obviously, this is only one possible line of exploration among various others, and only a first step along that line. Another possible way of beginning inquiries is to follow Freud's suggestion for help in understanding human situations: "Go to the poets." That is, the study of literary accounts of illness in a family context might offer leads and insights, much as such an approach has been useful at times in both psychiatric and anthropological studies of problematic behavior. But the particular method is not the main point; what matters is to take seriously the possible significance of interaction for illness, and to initiate exploratory inquiry based firmly on this viewpoint.

## Potential Benefits—And Some Caveats

Most of the direct potential benefits of the sort of work proposed here are rather obvious, or plainly implied in the earlier discussion of its rationale. Such work might lead to significant alterations and advances in our understanding of particular diseases that are important because of in their spread or severity. In turn, better understanding could lead to imply improvements in prevention and treatment, individually and more widely. It is worth noting, however, that the relationship between greater under standing and practical importance is apt to be complex and unpredictable For instance, the discovery of some interaction pattern that merely predisposes persons to a certain disease could be more readily applicable, and therefore practically important, than some more sweeping finding. The whole question of the economics of illness and its control, in the broadest sense, is involved here in much the same way as in public health generally. If various factors are seen to be involved in the onset and course of any disease, the problems of its costs and its control might correspondingly be attacked in various ways, focusing on one another, or several of the factors. There is no intrinsically best way; the approach of choice will depend on the existing knowledge, evaluations of the importance of the problem, and the given social context, which includes both available material resources and, not least, preferred modes of thinking and action about disease generally.

Such prospects are large, but also uncertain. It is certain that such inquiries and their application would require much difficult work. This would be difficult enough intrinsically, given its complexities and exploratory nature. It would be more difficult because it would be an attempt, both conceptually and practically, to make headway against the mainstream of current medicine—at the same time that some medical cooperation would be needed to carry it out.

If any such work were done, however, it would also contribute toward developing and promoting a broader and potentially more useful general conception of illness, essentially a behavioral or even ecological view of disease. In much the same way that we now increasingly see "mental illness" not as separate disorder but as ordered through unfortunate behavior, explainable in terms of interaction, we might contribute toward a view of disease that would diminish the separation of "pathology" from "health." Rather, both might be seen and seen better, as sorts of functioning to be understood in terms of interaction of the human organism with other humans, as well as with other sorts of organisms and with the inorganic environment.

To mention this possibility might appear to be suggesting a simple but grandiose inversion of the old imposition of the medical model on "mental illness," about which we have justifiably complained, but this is not the case. For one thing, the interactional viewpoint, based on cybernetics and systems theory, is inherently more general and comprehensive than the traditional medical model of illness and treatment. For another, I am not suggesting a takeover but an expansion or supplementing of medical views—and in a general direction some medical thinking is already struggling toward.

Still, such a broad interactional conception of illness would hardly be immediately and widely welcomed by the medical world. Yet it might gradually find some welcome and use. For one example, psychosomatic medicine already involves a related framework, but one that to a considerable extent is implicit, narrow, and piecemeal. A broader and more explicit interactional viewpoint could be useful there. For another, there is the newly-christened field of family medicine. Kellner (1963) and other perceptive physicians have in recent years observed and reported clusters and associations of illnesses occurring in families, and students are increasingly being trained in family medicine as a specialty. Yet so far, there appears to be no general framework in use to help these physicians go beyond simple noting of temporal association and sequence in interrelating such illnesses, or to help the students view in a unitary way the families whose members they are to treat. Our viewpoint might be useful here also, where a related need is unusually manifest.

Finally, we may conclude by considering the pursuit of the interactional viewpoint, beyond those areas where it is already established, in the widest perspective. That is, keeping in mind that throughout this paper we are not concerned with abstract truth, but with the utility of viewpoints—ways of observing and conceiving our experiential world, and their consequences –one may examine the prospects, positive and negative, that are inherent in the nature of the interactional viewpoint, as compared to other viewpoints.

Throughout history, both laymen and a variety of professionals have been concerned with examining and explaining human events, especially any kinds of events seen as difficult or problematic. Until recently, most such explanation has followed one of two general lines of thought. Human events and problems have often been seen as the outcome or consequence of powerful impersonal forces, external to the human realm. Such forces may be physical, social in a broad sense, or supernatural—such as climate or geography, economics or class structure, fate or God's will. To this list, in a modern and scientific age, one may add small yet powerful microbes and viruses. Or, human events and behavior have been explained as a consequence of intrinsic human factors—physical, mental or moral attributes seen as characteristic of individual persons or groups and determining their behavior. These two broad viewpoints appear to be very different, even polar. Yet like many polar opposites they have much in common at a more general level. Both lead toward considering the nature of any given situation or problem as evident, usually achieved either by the sharp division of problems into separate and discrete kinds, or lumping them into a global category, and focusing inquiry rather on their "why" or "who." Both lead toward an orientation to ultimate—primal causes or final solutions, or both. Both tend to place the locus of responsibility for problems and their handling beyond one's own human sphere, whether by attribution to nonhuman forces, or by labelling some other party as inherently bad or mad, and as causing the problem. Both easily lead either to resigned acceptance, or a call for the power of some higher authority, whether this be God, a leader, or science, to resolve matters.

The interactional viewpoint appears as rather new, as yet rather limited, and as very different from all this. It looks at human events and problems concretely various yet generally similar—primarily in terms of behavior occurring between persons in some system of social relationships. It assumes that the nature of difficulties often is *not* self-evident, and focuses inquiry on the "what" and "how" of the situation in question. Such inquiry is less concerned with ultimate origins or ends than with the present situation, how this is being maintained and how it might be altered for the better, though no solution will ever be final or perfect. Viewing of problems in relation to interaction also puts them on a human scale, and in terms of *joint* responsibility: "All in it together" rather than an "all or none or either you or me" responsibility of specific parties. This implies further that better problem handling is a joint enterprise, and potentially mutually beneficial, not mainly a matter of winners or losers.

It seems plain that it is this general interactional viewpoint that provides the main common bond among us, beyond our specific differences of idea and practice, and that has led us to a more human, behavioral, and useful understanding of "mental illness." This viewpoint, however, is general: it is not inherently restricted to mental or emotional problems. It might quite similarly, and perhaps as usefully, be applied to other problems, and specifically to illness. Yet, even if inquiry based on a similar viewpoint began to discern significant relationships between interaction and illness—in fact, perhaps especially then—a serious difficulty probably would arise. "We're all in it together" is a more humane and generally more useful view of problems than "We're right and he's wrong." Yet this is not the usual view, blame is more popular than sharing of responsibility, and as we know, people are seldom eager for change in their basic views.

This difficulty, of course, is not unfamiliar. We face it constantly in promoting the interactional viewpoint in our own work with families. But there we have some experience and methods of dealing with it; for physical illness, the situation would be new, and quite possibly more severe. Any positive findings about interaction and disease might well, at least initially, be seen more as accusations that people are making their loved ones sick than as a realistic and helpful recognition of how, without benefit of ceremony even, we are in life together, for better or worse, in sickness and in health, until death do us part—and sometimes even beyond. In the wider application of our interactional viewpoint, then, there is a prospect of progress, but no certainty except of hard work and conflict. Perhaps, after all, we should just mind our own business and not get involved.

## References

Bursten.(1965). Family Dynamics, the sick role, and medical hospital admissions, *Family Process* , 4, 206-216 (1965)

Cannon, W. (1920). *Bodily Changes in Pain, Hunger, Fear & Rage.* 2nd edition, New York: Appleton.

Cannon, W. (1942). Voodoo death, *American Anthropologist,* 44:169-81.

Dunbar, F. (1954). *Illness & Bodily Changes.* New York, Columbia University Press.

Haley, J. (1958). An Interactional Explanation of Hypnosis, *Amierican Journal of Clinical Hypnosis* 1, No. 2.41-57.

Herman, M. (1955, April 13). *A Critique of Psychosomatics.* Read at the Fifth Annual Institute in Psychiatry & Neurology, V.A. Hospital, Lyons, New Jersey.

Kellner, R. (1963). *Family Ill Health—An Investigation in General Practice.* NY, Thomas.

Meissner, W. (1966). Family dynamics & psychosomatic processes. *Family Process*, 5,142-161.

Shands, H. (1960). *Semiotic Approaches to Psychiatry.* The Hague, Mouton.

Selye, H. (1956). *The Stress of Life.* New York. McGraw-Hill.

Spark, C. & Brody, E. (1970). The aged are family members, *Family Process* 9, 195-210.

Grolnick, L. (1972). A Family Perspective of Psychosomatic Factors in Illness. A Review of the Literature, *Family Process* 11, 457-86.

# CHAPTER 8

# "Sometimes it's better for the right hand not to know what the left hand is doing"[1]

*Richard Fisch, M.D.*

Mrs. S. called me. She said her son needed help. He was 12 years old and was having trouble with other children at school and at home. She wasn't sure how to set up the appointment but would leave it to my decision. I asked her if her son would be resistant to coming in and she replied that she wasn't sure but that he had no trouble relating to adults. When she began to elaborate on that I told her it would be best to leave any further description of the problem till we met in my office. I further suggested that it might be better in the long run for me to meet only with her and her husband, at least for that first session. She was agreeable to that.

(I discourage patients from giving me much information on the phone. I do this because I want to convey that treatment is a "getting down to business," not a casual affair to be discussed over a phone. I also want to convey a separation between my office and their lives outside of it. This helps set the stage when, later in treatment, I may further convey that, while discussion may be needed, it is action in their lives that is more important. As for who to see

[1] Originally published in P. Papp (Ed.), (1977). *Family Therapy: Full Length Case Studies*, New York: Gardner Press.

in an initial session, this will often be determined by my assessment as to who, in the family, is the complainant and not, necessarily by who is the identified patient. In a child-centered problem, it is almost always the parents who are the complainants, not the child, and since they are also the power in the family, I usually anticipate I will be doing the greater bulk of the work with them. Thus, having the parents come in initially conveys that *they* are initiating treatment and are asking my help in *their* dealings with *their* child. On occasion, I may see the child with his or her parents in the first interview, but I will never see a child alone the first time.)

### *Session* 1.

Mr. and Mrs. S. arrived on time. She is thirty-seven years old and he thirty-eight. They are an attractive couple; both are slim, youthful and athletic looking. Both are engineers working in the electronics field, although Mrs. S's job is part-time. In addition to their 12-year-old son, Billy, they have an 8-year-old boy, Larry. Mrs. S. reiterated her concern about Billy.

The principal problem had to do with his difficulty in socializing with children, especially with those his own age. In school, he often got into fights and seemed to be generally hostile to the other children. The problem had reached its peak about two years ago when he got into a "rage reaction" at school and had to be sent home. While the problem had subsided some in the last two years, it was still considerable and treatment was precipitated by a recent call from his teacher; that he had had another "outburst" in class and was sent home for misbehavior at school, although not all of it for "outbursts" or "rage reactions." They added that Billy's difficulties were not limited to school. He had no friends in their neighborhood, either and he would spend "75 percent" of his time watching television. They would scold him for spending so much of his time in front of the TV set; would try to limit the hours of watching and urge him to go outside and meet with other children, but this was to no avail. When I asked how he got along with Larry, they said they frequently squabbled with each other but did not identify this as any particular problem; it was not excessive in their minds, did not reach uncontrollable levels, and it appeared to be a mutual bickering rather than any harassment by Billy, per se.

Then they launched into a rather pessimistic picture—Billy was "neurologically and physically handicapped." At about 4 or 5 years of age he was diagnosed as having psychomotor epilepsy and through the years had been maintained on anti-convulsive medications. This had markedly limited his seizures so that in the last year or two he had had only four episodes. These, they described, came on only at night and while he was asleep. However, he had also been diagnosed as having a "pore cephalic cyst" and that this lesion had left him with spasticity of the left hand. For this he had gone to physical therapy and while function had improved he still had noticeable spasticity and difficulty with fine touch movement. But this was not the end of his "neurological" problems. Later, during his schooling, he had been diagnosed by school personnel as having "dyslexia" and because of this diagnosis had been placed in special education classes for the last two years. It seemed that such placement was also determined by his hostile behavior in class and the decision to transfer him was precipitated by his "rage reaction" and the teacher fearing she could no longer control him. Finally, Mrs. S. said that because of all the problems Billy presented she had been able to look back and realize that from birth he was "hyperactive" and difficult to handle.

In asking for Mr. S.' views, he echoed much of what his wife had said. However, he added that Billy also suffered from some kind of frustration he was unable to put into words. They would often question him—"Why are you upset? What really bothers you?" And they would be dismayed when he responded in a self-denigrating way: "I always botch things up. Why is everything I do a boo-boo?" They attempted to help him by giving him "environmental support"—trying to find things for him to do he could feel good about himself in accomplishing, taking him on special trips skiing, golfing, bicycle riding, picnics. When the parents went out they made a special effort to find sitters who would be "supportive" such as male college students. They acknowledged this tended to limit their social life since such sitters were hard to come by. Finally, they would make "contracts" with Billy and give him special rewards for being a "nice kid."

(I made no comments throughout this narrative. My sole activity was to raise questions to clarify the points they were making: what they regarded as the problem, what had precipitated their decision to seek treatment, how they had attempted to deal with or help Billy overcome his problem and what kind of outcome of therapy they wanted. I had gotten a rather clear picture of the problem and how they had been attempting to "solve" it. My principal uncertainty was how to evaluate the neurological picture and how to find the leverage to deal with the parent's implicit pessimism about their son. As for the former, I was more concerned about the epilepsy and the spasticity than I was the "dyslexia." I do not regard "dyslexia," "minimal brain damage" or "learning disability" as valid or constructive ways of explaining a child's school difficulties. In addition, I know that these diagnoses can be very loosely used and are resorted to by some schools to protect their own educational philosophies of hidden coercion—much as "schizophrenia" is used to obscure parental or social agency mis-management. But I also knew that these parents had firmly accepted this definition of Billy's trouble and that this enlarged their pessimistic expectations of him. These expectations were then manifested in the numerous "helping" efforts they had described which had turned the school and the home into treatment centers for him and could, at the very least, only add to his one-down self-consciousness. I anticipated that, whatever else I would do, I would want to get the parents to move away from that position. I, therefore, anticipated with them that I might have to work with Billy through them, explaining to that since he had been subjected to such a profusion of special services it could be counter-productive for me to work with him directly while he struggled with the additional stigma of having to see a "shrink.")

Before ending the session, I said that as a next step I felt it important to see Billy but that after that I might ask to see them again. They were agreeable to that and we stopped.

(In seeing Billy, I had in mind to check out the report of his "gross neurological problem" as well as get my own appraisal of his general demeanor and his accounting for his difficulty with other children. Seeing him alone could have another use. Should I need some rationale for supporting any advice to the parents they might question, I could refer to "material" that presumably came up in the session with Billy, material that could not be challenged because of the privacy of the session and my own "expert" interpretation of that material.)

### Session 2. (Four days later.)

Billy was a pleasant looking boy and more outgoing than I had anticipated. He was slightly small for his age but in the course of discussion it never came up as a consideration on his part and did not seem to be any problem to him. I told him that his parents had seen me because they were concerned about his not having friends at school or at home. I asked him if this was a problem for him or were his parents being overly concerned? He appeared slightly uncomfortable in answering that question and said that he did have some friends at home. He acknowledged that he had no friends at school and did little with the friends he had at home, but on further elaboration about what he did do with his friends he implied that he had no dealings with them and that he did spend most of his free time watching television.

(I did not make any point of this "confession" nor confront him with it, but merely accepted his statements as helping me to be clearer on things. With children, as with adults, initial sessions are devoted to data seeking and are conducted matter-of-factly but with specific questions designed to elicit special information. My principal goal at that stage is to get a clear, concise picture of the significant transactions in the patients' lives, especially those revolving around the problem. Also, I am always looking for "leverages"—what is important and meaningful to the patient which I can use to get them to accept suggestions from me; suggestions which redefine a situation or ones which influence them to take some necessary action in their lives and regarding their problem. Since my highest priority is on action and little or none on "insight," "confrontation" plays a minimal role in my therapy.)

I shifted in my questioning. I said that while his parents might be concerned about his not having friends, it might not be of any concern to him; was there something different *he* was concerned about. He readily answered that his biggest complaint was that he has been "bugged all my life." He explained that he has been made fun of and harassed about his left hand. I told him that his parents had mentioned his left hand to me but that I would appreciate it if he would show me what kind of trouble he had with it. He then demonstrated by slowly and jerkily picking up a nearby ashtray, holding it between his thumb and forefinger and explaining while he did so how much trouble he was having and that I should notice how his "fingers didn't work right." I moved my chair closer to his and watched with apparent curiosity as he performed this spastic task. When he put the ashtray down, I told him that I found that a very intriguing way to pick up the ashtray and would he please show me again just how he did that. He seemed pleased to oblige me and as he repeated the task I made my own comments on the complexity of movements required by his hand and fingers to be *able* to pick it up in just that fashion. I asked him to perform other tasks with his hand and marveled, each time, at the way his hand performed it. Then I began trying to imitate his hand's movements but I always failed and expressed frustration that I couldn't do with my hand what he so easily could do with his left hand. He was surprised at my failure and this allowed me to tell him that I would bet his father couldn't do it either. When he challenged this I said, "I'll tell you what. I bet that even your right hand can't imitate your left." He tried, but as I anticipated, he was unable to do it. For some moments, then he looked at his left hand wonderingly and admiringly.

(Since for him, perhaps not his parents, the most meaningful problem was focused on his left hand, I decided to see what I could do with that. I had not anticipated this before seeing him nor even in the earlier part of the session. But since I always looking to use whatever is thrown my way I began to formulate a way of working with his hand to redefine his one-down position to a one-up. I began this redefinition by expressing interested curiosity in his hand, then by referring to its spastic movements as worthy of further, greater attention then by referring to the movements as an *ability,* and finally as an ability that was unique and implicitly superior to those of mine, his father and even his stronger hand. His response to that indicated his acceptance of the redefinition and rather than labor the point, I shifted to a slightly different area.)

I asked him, as if it were a new and sudden thought, "Are there any kids at school who *don't* bug you about your hand?" He said there were. I said, "You know, you don't have to just wait for some kid to bug you, you can be in charge of some of the bugging." Since he appeared intrigued by that thought, I challenged him to see if he could pick out one kid who had never bugged him and, *without saying a word,* see if he could get that kid to bug him about his hand. He was quite agreeable, almost gleeful about the idea and we ended the session on that note.

(I was assuming that Billy's apprehension about being "bugged" would, through his defensive and withdrawn posture, invite harassment and recreate a self-fulfilling prophecy. I was, therefore, attempting to interdict that cycle by getting him to be *curious* about the "bugging" and, at the same time, even less defensive by defining it as something he could control—not simply be victimized by.)

### Session 3. (Six days later.)

Mr. and Mrs. S. came at my request. I said that I had had a most instructive and enlightening session with Billy. They commented that something of some significance must have happened since he had gone around for several days after showing them what he could do with his left hand. Before, he had tended to keep it hidden. I told them I had shown great curiosity in his hand but I expressed surprise that it had made such an impact on him. In passing, I attributed this welcome change in Billy to their innate curiosity and patience.

(When I have had any beneficial impact on a child, I attempt to minimize my own influence and, instead, attribute progress to some quality or effort of the parents. I always want to strengthen the idea that it is *their* ability to positively influence their child and, thereby, enhance their optimism and willingness to take further steps.)

I told them that in that session I was able to get a handle on what might be underlying Billy's poor self-esteem, his unhappiness and, therefore, his a-socialization. I explained that with his disability and all the years of doctors' appointments, treatments, special programs and the attention that has surrounded his difficulties he had become fearful of being in the omnipotent position of reordering his parents' lives; that while he had some concern about his own possible fragility, he was more concerned that his parents were too fragile and intimidated by him and his disability and that he was in control. This fear, I continued, held him back from risking approaching other children. As could be seen, all their well meant urgings, encouragements, special outings, and the like, were seen by Billy as evidences of their intimidation and he was unable to profit from them.

(The above explanation to the parents regarding Billy's "fear of omnipotence" is an example of a type of framing I often find necessary. In this case I had already formed some general idea of what I wanted the parents to do, principally to stop the well meant campaign of intrusiveness in his life through their questioning, exhortations, "special programs" and the like. I believed that all that could only add to his self-consciousness and therefore his difficulty m socializing.

However, it is one thing to know what the parents should do, it is another to get them to do it. I could have simply told them what I believed, that he is essentially a normal boy despite his left-handed motor problem but a boy made self-conscious by their well intended help. But this would have run counter to all their beliefs about him; they saw the problem as starting almost from birth, over the years their lives revolved more and more around his problem and they viewed him as having deficits—neurologically and psychologically—that set him apart from other normal children; To have ignored their views would have run the risk of their discounting any further input I could provide and, worse, set them to seek a more pathology-oriented therapist for their son. Thus, I felt it necessary to frame any further advice by an explanation which incorporated their own belief system but with some elaboration of my own that would make any ensiling suggestions "logical" in their minds.

In its essence, they were seeing Billy as having some significant psychological problem which led him to have a poor image of himself and in-turn contributing to his difficulty making friends. Since I was the "expert" I was then free to describe what, in my "expertise" had come to light regarding the exact nature of that psychological problem. It was not too difficult to refer to "a fear of omnipotence." I had reason to use that framing before *for* parents who needed to treat their child matter-of-factly, at times punitively, but who were intimidated by the notion the child was "mentally ill" or "sick." To tell parents, then, that their child's "sickness" requires a departure from "egg-shell" handling allows them to shift more easily to a matter-of-fact management. In this case, as in many cases, the parents are overly conscientious and this reframing also allows them something to do *for* their child. In any case, it is more certain that people will back off from some traditional position if they are given something to do that requires a 180 degree shift.)

They said this made a lot of sense but confirmed their own suspicions that they were not handling Billy right. Since their implied sense of ineptness might interfere with their getting on with what they needed to do I said that most of what they had done for Billy was necessary and should not have been different and that I was commenting on those few things that might not, at this point, be useful to continue. In any case, what they did was born from their sincere desire to help him and for most children would be logical. Since they seemed to relax on hearing that I proceeded to detail what they now could do.

I reminded them that what I was about to suggest might still seem strange, but they were to keep in mind that it stemmed from my awareness of Billy's need to overcome his feared omnipotence. To begin with there needed to be a separation between Billy's world at school and his world at home; that whatever difficulties he had at school should not intrude itself into the activities and routines of his parents. Therefore, the school should be notified that whatever problems they encountered with Billy were to be handled by them and under no circumstances should he be sent home for any misbehavior. I said that it would help the school authorities relax if they were also told they could use their own judgment in handling Billy in any way they deemed appropriate. In keeping with this, I further suggested that they not punish him for any delinquencies that occurred at school; this would not only avoid reduplicated penalties but, more importantly, convey to him that he is not in a position any longer to "force" them to go out of their way to impose disciplinary measure simply by acting up at school. Finally, I asked them that they not only discontinue urging him to get out of the house and make friends but that they actively discourage it. I suggested this might best be done by telling them that they prefer he stay home as much as possible since it's easier to keep track of him and avoids the possibility of his bringing home some noisy children. Instead, he could "watch those nice shows on TV." Mrs. S. agreed quite readily and seemed to sense some humor in it. She smiled and said, "Well, at least that will be some switch." However, Mr. S., while agreeing to the plan, expressed concern that Billy might simply follow their instructions. I said that was possible, but since they had already made a concerted effort to get him out of the house with no success, there was nothing to lose by shifting tack. I added that what I was suggesting might not initially aid Billy's socialization, but that it was directed to a first or more basic step, their conveying to him that his friendlessness was not a burden to them. This seemed to reassure Mr. S. and we ended the session with the plan to meet in two weeks.

(As the reader can tell, all these suggestions and comments were designed to aid the parents in backing away from a management of their son which I felt could only be confirming and adding to his self-consciousness and difficulty in socializing. In effect, I was attempting to get them to stop *creating* a problem. For further elaboration of this rationale, the reader is referred to *Change—Principles of Problem Formation and Problem Resolution* by Watzlawick, Weakland and Fisch, W. W. Norton (1974).

### Session 4. (Twelve days later.)

When they came in, Mrs. S. began right away saying that they had done what I asked and a few days later Billy had brought home two friends. She laughed as she said that he had even made lunch for them and she didn't mind the mess he had made in the kitchen. He hadn't repeated that since but she expressed amazement that their new tack would have such rapid and definite results. I expressed amazement also; that while I had hoped for some sign of less tension on Billy's part, I was surprised that it went further and I indicated that I was disconcerted that improvement had gone so fast.

(When patients or parents come in and announce a definite improvement, an improvement they are clearly acknowledging, I am most likely going to take the position that "things have moved too fast" and that, therefore, no further improvement should take place "for the time being." I may offer various rationales for this position but most often will simply say that in my experience, there is more danger changing things too fast than too slow. There is little, if any, error in this strategy since it is my general view that problems are more likely to arise when people are working too hard at things rather than at a leisurely pace. While patients are encouraged by initial success, it is too easy for them to become apprehensive lest the improvement isn't sustained. Their intensified and urgent efforts can often be counter-productive and produce a demoralizing retrogression. If, on the other hand, their therapist looks a bit worried about the unexpected efficiency of their efforts, it underscores the potential for change and, at the same time puts them in the more relaxed position of not having to keep up the effort. Often, I may not only suggest that things should not improve further, but I will suggest that they make an effort to have things slide back a "peg or two." Thus, should any retrogression occur, this is not demoralizing since it is "according to plan." In actuality, it is rare for things to retrogress, and more often than not patients come in and smilingly tell me they had "failed" in their efforts to hold things back.)

They also reported that the school was quite willing to cooperate with their request, in fact almost seemed relieved. They said they couldn't add much more since "things have been quiet" on the school front since then. As we were about to end Mr. S. said that they had been planning to send Billy to a special school for dyslexic children sometime in the fall and what did I think about that. I attempted to discourage it by saying that while it might be necessary this school semester had just begun and there wasn't enough time to evaluate Billy's potential for progress; that it might be better to wait further. I added that while such a special school could have its advantages in meeting some of Billy's needs, it would have the disadvantage of gearing his educational experience even further away from the more regular context than the special classes he was in. This could have a bearing on the very problem they were coming in about, his difficulty in socialization and the marginal position he has been in vis-a-vis other children. I then asked that we meet again in about three weeks.

### Session 5. *(Three weeks later.)*

Mrs. S. came in by herself. She said that her husband had wanted to come in but since he was starting a new job they both felt it best he not take too much advantage of working hours. She said that Billy was "still holding his own." He had had friends over again, was spending more of his time out of the house and consequently less time watching television. She also reported that one morning when he had missed the school bus he simply took his bicycle and got himself to school. She regarded that as significant since characteristically he would ask her to drive him to school. She said he is still reluctant to attend school and she feels it necessary to get him up in the morning, urge him to speed up in getting ready so he won't miss the bus and the like. I suggested that his slowness in preparing for school was another facet of the overall problem—his fear that his own difficulties could push the parents around, and that it could be dealt with as they had done with the school and his getting out of the house after school. I therefore suggested that at least on one morning she make an effort to get him to be late and we discussed some ways of implementing that—not setting the alarm, being slow in serving breakfast, etc. However, I told her that while I thought this might be helpful to him, on second thought, it might be taking things a little too fast again. I wasn't sure so she should think it over but not feel she should rush into it, beneficial as it might be. I ended the session and, again, suggested we meet in three weeks.

(As mentioned previously, I feel there is more danger in attempting to move patients on after there has been a report of improvement than in taking the position of "go slow." At the very worst, should I underestimate the confidence of the patient in moving ahead, he will make it clear to me that he is quite impatient and the impetus *for* change will all the more come *from* him. Therefore, while Mrs. S. was describing another facet of Billy's problem, she was defining it as a lesser one and the previous improvement he had shown was still holding up. I felt it important not to press it further but to appear to withdraw my suggestion. In implying that it would, nevertheless, be a beneficial move, I could allow her to go ahead with it but in a relaxed way since I was attaching no importance or urgency to it.)

### Session 6. *(Three weeks later.)*

Mr. and Mrs. S. came in together. Mrs. S. said that Billy was coming along fine, especially with friends. His contacts with children in the neighborhood were now more and more frequent and there had evolved some visiting at each other's houses. She seemed quite pleased but Mr. S., while acknowledging those gains, looked uncomfortable and tense. He expressed concern that, while things seemed to be going well, they might not be *fully* attending to

Billy's needs, for example, his need to be more responsible. On further exploration, it turned out that Billy's "irresponsibilities" were minimal and Mr. S. acknowledged that they weren't any problem. He explained that the *real* problem for him was his anxiety that they weren't doing their best; that he was not carrying out my suggestions *correctly* and that they were making mistakes that would show up sooner or later. Since Mrs. S. didn't seem bothered by this, I directed my comments to her husband. I told him that since Billy's trouble had as one element a lack of confidence, it would be greatly beneficial if his father could convey that by making mistakes himself even in his handling of Billy. This might now be his most beneficial effort with Billy, while his wife could continue the previous tack we had discussed. Therefore, I urged him to make sure he made some mistakes with Billy, at least from "time to time." He relaxed on hearing that and I concluded the session by saying that I felt we should meet in two weeks.

(On hearing the mother's report, that gains in Billy's socialization had been maintained, even elaborated on, I anticipated that this might be a terminating session. While the reader may well feel this is a rather precipitous, I believe there are fewer risks in terminating treatment after a small, but strategic, change has occurred. Billy's a-socialization had been a rather long-standing business and in a matter of a short space of time he had done quite well. The leap from no friends to one friend is a much greater one than from one friend to two friends. Much of the business of doing therapy briefly is knowing what *not* to meddle with. However, the father's reaction discouraged me from bringing up the offer of termination. I therefore decided to redefine his "incorrectness" as a therapeutically beneficial and necessary feature of the overall treatment. Although he showed some visible relaxation following that, I thought it would help to plan the next session sooner than we had been accustomed to.)

### Session 7. *(Two weeks later.)*

Mr. and Mrs. S. came in and said that things were going quite well with Billy. Both were visibly pleased. Neither could think of any complaints about his deportment and as far as they could tell analogous improvement had taken place *in* the school setting. They said that they had some unexpected trouble, not from Billy, but from his brother, Larry. He had taken some money from a younger child. On learning of it they had taken him over to that child's home, had him apologize to the boy and his parents, return the money and, after some brief discussion with the boy's parents, took Larry back home.

Again, Mr. S.' main concern was not that Larry was becoming a problem, but wondering whether they had handled the incident thoroughly and correctly enough. Since I felt they had handled it quite well, I limited my comments to predicting that the only error I could be sure they would make at any time in the future would be to underestimate their beneficial handling of situations that arose with the kids. I would never fear they hadn't done enough, only that they would never feel they had. They acknowledged that this had been an old Achilles heel of theirs, especially his. Mrs. S. then said she felt confident enough about the kids and their handling of them that she was planning to quit her part-time job and divert her time to endeavors of a more leisurely sort; things she had been looking forward to for many years.

I then took the opportunity of suggesting that we either stop treatment or, at least, take a long vacation from it. They said they were really quite pleased, even amazed, at the progress Billy had made and they preferred to stop treatment at this point; perhaps leave things ad hoc should anything come up.

### Follow up. (Two months later.)

Mrs. S. called and said that things had been going quite well. Billy was doing fine in school, not getting into fights, making friends there as well as in the neighborhood. They were having no further trouble with Larry. She added that she and her husband were quite pleased with the outcome of treatment and thanked me for "what almost seems a miracle." I said that I appreciated their thanks and that while I needed all the credit I could get, I knew they deserved a major portion of it for the efforts they had made, the willingness to try out some "crazy stuff" and the way they went about it. I promised her, though, that since I did need the credit, I wouldn't divulge to anyone that they had had any part in Billy's improvement. Mrs. S. recognized my facetiousness and we ended the telephone conversation.

(As I mentioned in the opening of this case, I always want to convey that it's the parents' child and their effort that will count. I do not back away from this position because a case has gone well or has terminated. In my final rejoinder on the phone, I simply used humor, to convey that message.)

# CHAPTER 9

# "OK-You've Been a Bad Mother."

## *John H. Weakland*

My specific ideas, actions, and reactions in dealing with this case—involving a 15-year-old-boy with school and behavior problems as the identified patient and his divorced parents—can only be understood in relation to their context, the general approach developed at the Brief Therapy Center of the Mental Research Institute over the past ten years. The basic ideas and procedures involved in this approach have been described at some length elsewhere (Weakland, Fisch, Watzlawick, & Bodin, 1974; Watzlawick, Weakland, & Fisch, 1974). Here, I hope a brief summary of these will be adequate for orientation to the case material to follow, which in turn may clarify the general approach by concrete illustration of its application.

How one conducts therapy—and evaluates the outcome—depends greatly on one's general view of the nature of problems. In common with other family therapists our Center views problems as interactional—that is, not something residing in a particular individual, but an aspect or a resultant of interaction between individuals in a family, or in some other ongoing system of social interaction and communication. Along with this, we view problems as behavioral in nature—that is, as consisting of behavior by the identified patient, which is stimulated and shaped by behavior of other persons involved (or sometimes by other behavior of the patient himself). Accordingly, we see

[1] Originally published in P. Papp (Ed.), (1977). *Family Therapy: Full Length Case Studies*, New York: Gardner Press.

problem resolution as requiring behavioral changes by those involved in the system of interaction, and the essential business of the therapist as one of promoting such change, which the members of the system have not been able to accomplish on their own. These views too are common enough among family therapists. We differ from many family therapists however, in our concentration on the presenting problem, in our focus of intervention and our goal of treatment, and in our means of promoting change. For the most part, these differences rest upon pursuing the interactional view of problems. in concept and practice, further than is commonly done-even when our practice appears oriented to one individual.

If one really focuses on behavior, any problem—of the kind people bring to therapists—may he defined generally as consisting of (a) some observable behavior, which (b) is characterized as undesirable (distressing, difficult, deviant) either by its performer or by some other concerned person, but which (c) persists despite efforts to get rid of it. Accordingly, our treatment begins by inquiring what the problem is, in behavioral terms—what is the identified patient doing and saying that constitutes a problem. This includes, unless it is obvious, how this constitutes a problem. That is, we see the behavior as itself the problem, not as "the tip of the iceberg," the outer sign of more fundamental inner feelings, nor even necessarily a manifestation of some deep and pervasive disarray in the system of interaction. On this basis, we next inquire not about the nature of interaction as a whole in a family, but about behavior immediately related to the problem behavior—namely, what is being done to try to handle (prevent or resolve) the problem by the identified patient or others concerned.

Both a general view and concrete experience underlie this focus. The interactional view of problems implies a cybernetic rather than a linear concept of causation. On this view, not the origin but the persistence of a problem is central for understanding and treatment (Maruyama, 1963; Wender, 1968). That is, what behaviors function to maintain or reinforce the performance of the problem behavior, although this is defined as undesired or undesirable? Ironically, in our experience it regularly appears that while people's attempts to handle the existing problem usually are well-intentioned and often apparently logical, something in them constitutes the reinforcing behavior: "The 'solution' is the problem."

In other words, problems consist most basically of vicious circles, involving a positive feed-back loop between some undesired behavior and inappropriate efforts to get rid of it. In our approach several things follow from this view. Our general treatment aim is to interrupt the vicious circle maintaining the problem behavior. Our specific interventions are therefore aimed primarily at interdicting the misguided solution being pursued. This often may involve the substitution of some other opposite or incompatible behavior, but this is a means of insuring change, not the essential change itself. Also, an apparently small but strategic change in problem handling may serve to initiate a beneficent circle leading to progressive further improvement, so that long-term treatment and heroic changes are not required.

In making such interventions, since our aim is behavioral change rather than intellectual understanding—which in family therapy as in individual treatment may produce no change in actual daily behavior—we do not devote much effort to clarifying and describing the interactional situation to those involved. Instead, we depend most on behavioral prescription, and on reframing the situation so as to make different problem-handling seem logical and appropriate to the participants, in terms of their own pre-existing ideas about people and problems. Finally, since we take the idea of interaction in systems seriously, we believe that it is possible to influence an entire system through appropriate change in any member. Therefore, rather than always seeing all the members of a family, we often concentrate our treatment attention and effort on whoever seems most ready for change, or possesses the greatest leverage in the system.

## The Z Case

I first heard of Jacky Z by a phone call from his mother. She told me that Jacky was doing poor work in school and being truant, as well as being difficult to handle at home, and both his high school counselor and the learning disability teacher in the special school he attended two days a week suggested me to her as a family counselor.

On the phone, Mrs. Z did not go into the specific difficulties much, but filled me in on the family background, which she saw as involving possible obstacles to treatment. Mr. and Mrs. Z had been divorced for 4 years, Mrs. Z having legal custody of the children. (Jacky at 15 was the youngest of three teen-age children. His older sister and older brother were described as no problem, and I never saw either of them.) The father had remarried shortly after the divorce, but still lived in the area, and maintained some contact with the children, however, Mrs. Z described him as a proud and rather stubborn man who had not been keen on the idea of family counseling when she had called him about it.

On hearing this, I told her that, while I would be glad to see Mr. Z also, for the way I work this would not be essential, at least to start with, and if he were urged he might well become more resistant. Therefore, I suggested, she might call him and say she was coming to consult me about Jacky and would be glad to have him come too if he wished, but she should avoid any appearance of pressing him. She sounded receptive to this, and said she would do so, and call me soon about a time to meet—since she wanted to leave this open to fit his schedule also. A few days later she called again, to report the whole situation had changed. When she called Mr. Z and made the proposal, his response was that no family counseling was needed, because the main problem was just that she wasn't handling Jacky right. Therefore, he would have Jacky come to live with him, and would soon have him squared away. Mrs. Z, apparently at her wits' end in trying to deal either with her son or his father, had agreed to give this a trial.

Reviewing this phone call, I had two thoughts. First, that I should have called Mr. Z myself, rather than leaving this to her. This, in fact, is what I would ordinarily do. I do not have any note as to why I did not in this case, so I cannot lie positive but it is highly likely that I was not especially eager to see the father anyway. Since the boy was living with his mother, I saw her as the key figure, and since she had seemed very receptive to my initial suggestions, I was confident I would be seeing her in any event. Second, that this confidence was a mistake; in all probability, Mrs. Z had not approached Mr. Z as I had suggested, and certainly she had acceded to a course of action different from what we had agreed on without consulting me. It will be evident later that I should have kept this indication that her readiness to agree did not mean equal readiness to act accordingly more in mind. But I did not, probably because after this call I mentally wrote off the inquiry as one of those things that might have been, but didn't develop.

Quite a few months later, though, I was surprised to get another call from Mrs. Z. She said that his father had not got Jacky squared away; instead, things were worse, including lots of difficulty between father and son, and Mr. Z was now willing to give counseling a trial. I made an appointment to meet with the two of them, stating that it would be desirable to get the basic information on the situation from them before seeing Jacky himself.

When they arrived, because of the previous phone contact and the lapse of time, I began by asking "What is the problem *now?*" I addressed this question first to Mrs. Z, since she had been the prime mover in instituting treatment. She began by reporting an incident that apparently was the precipitating event for seeking me out again. About a month before, Jacky did not return home to his father's house one evening. Instead, he called and said he was at his mother's house. But he was not; in fact, he did not show up at either house all night. Next day at school, the counselor found out that he had stayed over night with a friend. Since then, he had been coming home late on other occasions, and cutting school. Mrs. Z also said, more generally, that at the time Jacky went to live with his father he was completely out of her control. I asked "In what way?" to get more concrete behavioral information. She replied that he was also cutting school then, also he was smoking pot, and he had stolen and dismantled a bicycle. Also, without my asking, she volunteered some information on how she was trying to handle all this, saying "When I ask him: what's the matter, why does he do these things, I don't get an answer—he just doesn't communicate." This remark started me thinking that probably Mrs. Z was doing too much asking, in ways which defined her position as weak and ineffective, rather than telling her son what she expected of him, and taking some appropriate action to ensure compliance. I made a note of this, but no comment, at the time.

I then asked Mr. Z what the problem was, in his view. His style of response was positive and definite—only his statements were varied and contradictory: At the time of the bike theft, he had asked for Jacky to come and live with him, because "I've always felt he needs a man's company." Moreover, the school counselor had reported that once Jacky broke down and said "I never see my father." So, "Maybe Jacky felt abandoned by me. But, when I try to, he won't talk to me about it." On another front, Mr. Z reported that Jacky had been noted to be hyperactive in school some time ago. He had been put on Ritalin. However, some of the kids teased him about this ("You're taking dope") and recently the doctor had said Jacky has reached an age where he needs to learn self-control, not medication. Mr. Z also said Jacky is only doing third grade work, has no interest, can't sit still, is small for his age and people treat him like a baby; he has bad companions and no sense of responsibility. Mr. Z also said that Jacky doesn't talk, just keeps everything inside. But when Mrs. Z apparently agreed with this—"When I ask him if he knows what's right and wrong, he just answers 'Yes' and has no more to say" —Mr. Z then said "He's not just silent, he's full of excuses." This concluded the initial session, which I felt was rather emotional and chaotic, full of anger, anxiety and confusion, despite my attempts to structure it according to plan.

On reviewing this session a few days later, however, both the problem and its handling appeared clear enough, at least in main outline. Jacky was behaving badly both at school and at home, with acts both of omission and commission. Both father and mother were trying to handle this mainly by talk. Since each of them seemed to alternate frequently between the view "He's bad" and the view "He's sick," this talk similarly alternated between lectures and anxious inquiries, with the later probably predominating. They were persisting in such talk although it was getting nowhere—Jacky giving minimal answers and obvious excuses. Also, though this point was not really clear to me at the time, this persistence probably was being reinforced by the school counselor and learning disability teacher, who were indicating that Jacky had problems, that communication was the answer to this, and that Jacky did talk to *them*.

A week after the first session, Mrs. Z called to tell me that Mr. Z had backed out again ("He's always been leery of psychologists"), and—in obvious contrast to his "Let me handle things" stance—had asked her to call and cancel the second appointment that we had set up. Added to this was a report, though, that he had gotten firmer with Jacky, and the boy was behaving better now. My impression of her call was that she really felt powerless—that nothing could be done without Mr. Z's active cooperation—but was trying to maintain a hopeful stance: He's taking charge and Jacky's better. My own view was quite different, but I try not to argue with the client. I therefore told Mrs. Z, "Mr. Z does not have any full veto power over the therapy; some useful things by way of review and considering what may come next can be done without him. However, I can readily understand that you might feel like relaxing for a while. Jacky seems better right now, even if this should prove only temporary—and to go on now would mean acting without Mr. Z, perhaps even in some opposition to him. So think it over, take your time; you can always call me if you want to talk further."

At that point, while I certainly thought the Z's needed help, given the difficulties already encountered, I was quite uncertain if I would hear further from them. However, I also thought that to take the tack just described, of apparently backing off rather than pressing for a further meeting, would maximize the probability of further contact. I had my doubts as succeeding weeks went by, but in about a month Mrs. Z at last called me again. She reported that Jacky had been having further school difficulties, had been cutting school, and was finally suspended. His father had now agreed to cooperate further, though somewhat reluctantly. The main thing they had in mind, though, seemed to be that "Jacky might talk to you; he won't open up to either of us." This struck me as a further example of the idea "Communication is the answer," which I doubted as already noted, plus some note of "Fix him up and then send him back." However, I did want to get on with treatment, there was nothing to be lost by seeing Jacky and perhaps something to be gained by first-hand observation, even though I believed that from the parents' descriptions and my experience with similar problems I already had a rather reliable image of the boy. Therefore, I told Mrs. Z, "I don't know if he'll talk to me, but let's see. You bring him in—there's no use at this point, when it's not essential, to draw on Mr. Z's limited store of cooperation."

When Mrs. Z arrived with Jacky, I thought that he looked about like any 15-year-old boy, except that he was rather guarded in manner. I began by asking him "What's your understanding of why you're here?" He did not reply immediately, and after only a very brief silence his mother—always a rather nervously quick woman—began to press him: "Go on, answer the doctor, Jacky." This plainly irritated him and made him more reluctant to talk, but finally he said "I don't go to school, but no problem outside it." Within moments, mother and son were involved in a running argument: "You and my father always hassle me." "That is not so, you have a lot of freedom." "No, I don't." "You were getting into a lot of trouble, so something had to be done: I'm trying to explain why you were sent to live with your father." Very quickly the pattern was plain, and consistent with my expectation from the initial session: The boy makes brief complaints or accusations (or just silently looks pained), the mother responds with lengthy, defensive explanation or argument, and so on and on around the circle.

A small sample of this seemed plenty, so I asked Mrs. Z to wait while I talked with Jacky alone. My ideas in doing this were (a) it would be easier than having more redundant argument, (b) it would help my standing with Mrs. Z by complying with her expressed wish that I talk with him, and increase credence for any recommendations I might later make about dealing with him, and (c) though I had in mind working primarily with her, some useful intervention might be made directly with him. Once we were alone, I found that when asked a plain question and given a little time, he was reasonably forthcoming with answers. I began by asking if he thought he had any problems. "Just school—it's a drag. I don't want to go, but I have to." For the rest of the session, I deliberately took a stance as much as possible opposite to what I felt sure everyone else must have told him, over and over. First, I suggested that he really didn't *have* to go to school; people might threaten or exhort him, but they couldn't actually do much. I asked if he thought he had a learning disability. He said no, plainly, and went on to say he was getting C's as it is, and could get A's if he really tried. I suggested that probably he shouldn't, at least not anytime soon: since both his parents and teachers thought he has a learning disability, his getting A's would confuse and rattle them too much. He also mentioned that his parents' hassling him was a pain. I agreed, and asked how he handled this. He said "I try to do what they ask." I pointed out this might be a difficult, or perhaps impossible task, since it seemed to me that their demands might be unclear, inconsistent, and conflicting. He agreed. I wondered if he might make some headway in such circumstances by apparent agreement; that is, by saying, "Yes, yes" to whatever they asked. He gave it some thought, but was uncertain. I thanked him for coming, and sent him out, saying that we probably would meet again later, if only to help cool his parents' concern and hassling some by putting on the right appearance. In my thinking, this was both a further intervention—the opposite of "You've got big problems, and really need therapy"—and laying some ground work for getting him to come in readily if I should wish to see him again later. But I never did.

Mrs. Z was to call me about a further appointment, but again it was about a month before I heard from her. She had, however, been in the hospital for a minor operation during part of this time. She reported that Jacky was back with her; Mr. Z had thrown up his hands on dealing with him. Mrs. Z said that Jacky was all right—except that he was cutting school, smoking pot, stealing, and driving her up the wall. She raised the idea of a private school for him. Or, along the same line, what about sending him to summer camp—only the likely ones are full of his pot smoking friends. At this point, I realized that while I had gained a rather definite view of the problem and what kept it going, so far as treatment and change were concerned we had mainly been going around in circles, and seemed about to continue with more of the same. I therefore interrupted her to say that I understood from what she was saying that the problem still existed, and was quite serious—in fact, so serious that I thought it would be a mistake to try to give her any advice off the cuff in a phone conversation. Instead I proposed that I should review and think over the whole matter, and then call her back in a few days with some better recommendation on what should be done.

I did go through such a review, focusing my thinking mainly on how I might get her more firmly involved in treatment and more ready to follow any advice I wanted to give her on how to deal with Jacky more effectively. I then called her, and began by reemphasizing the serious and difficult nature of the situation. Since this was something she herself had been saying in various ways here and there, I assumed she would agree strongly with my statement, which proved correct. On similar grounds, I next stated that on the basis of my review of the problem, it appeared quite clear that as Jacky's mother she herself was the only one sufficiently concerned and influential to be in a position to give Jacky the help he needed so much—not his father, the school personnel, or even myself; though I would offer some advice, I was not important to Jacky and she was. Then, to block her from backing away from the problem again, I said that even though she was the only one in a position to really help Jacky, since he had given her a long hard time, I certainly could understand if she wanted to wash her hands of him instead. Mrs. Z, as I had hoped, responded "No, I'm confused and struggling, but I'm still ready. I'd like to get clearer how to deal with Jacky." I suggested that then it would be most appropriate for just the two of us to meet, and talk about that specifically; she agreed readily.

When she came in, I had one specific aim in mind: To get her to stop getting involved in defensive arguments with Jacky. Hoping to locate a specific initial target area for such change, I began by asking about her priorities—what was the main current difficulty, or what would she most like to see changed in Jacky's behavior. Her answers, however, were rather lengthy and rambling. She mentioned that he was going to school but not to classes, that she wanted to establish better communication, also more cooperation, but at one time he might talk and be helpful, then at another be silent and just do as he pleased. I attempted to shift the framing of "communication" from talk toward action by asking "Am I correct that at least part of the communication problem is that you can't tell what to expect from Jacky?" She agreed, and I went on to suggest that the basic problem seemed to be that Jacky needed to learn to be more responsible for his own behavior.

Then, in order to get more information on her own views—her "language" as we usually call it—I asked, "What is your best guess as to the reason for Jacky's behavior problem?" She said that there had been a lot of fighting between herself and Mr. Z at the time of divorce, repeated the report from the school counselor that Jacky had complained "I never see my father," and wondered if her involvement with another man had had an impact on Jacky. Almost at once, though, she went on to a different theme, "I really feel Jacky wants discipline."

Since this last remark was in line with my own thinking, I picked up on it immediately by saying "It does sound like things go a bit better when you say what you want from him more flatly, without much discussion or argument— and it might go still better if you could even be somewhat arbitrary." But, since I now was anticipating that she would probably retreat after any move toward taking more firm charge with Jacky, I went on to add "I don't really expect that, though. You are very frustrated by his behavior, but your hands are tied because you are carrying the blame for his problem."

At this, Mrs. Z burst into tears and said "I want a life of my own, but I have to supervise him." I considered that this ratified the picture of the situation I had been formulating on the basis of her answer to my question about her view of the cause of the problem—that Mrs. Z was feeling very guilty toward Jacky, and this got in the way of her taking more effective measures in handling him; therefore I needed to deal with this before anything else could be done.

To do so, I then took the steps which, in my estimation, constituted the turning point in the therapy. First I said "As I see it, the most important question is not the past, but where do we go from here." She agreed. I went on "However, the past is important, in that it keeps getting in the way because it remains unsettled. You may be taking on too much of the responsibility, because Mr. Z and the school people and even Jacky himself may be responsible in part for his problems. But I don't see *any* way to ever judge reliably just how much blame and responsibility really belongs to everyone involved. So, in order to get this over with, suppose we do like lawyers do on some issues and just stipulate 'It was *all* your fault.' She agreed to this, but with the beginning of a smile. "All right, *now* you are the crucial one if Jacky is to change."

Mrs. Z asked, "But how do you get through to a kid like that?" To me, this signaled a small but critical shift away from the problem itself, and the "why" of it, toward how to take useful action on it. This was confirmed when she went on to report an action she had already taken. "Jacky is still coming home late at times—but I've stopped going out to look for him." I replied "OK, but I don't know whether you could take the next step—if he is out late after you've asked him to be in by a certain time, lock up the house and go to bed at that time; then when he arrives, let him wait a while, finally let him in, and apologize for forgetting he was out." "I *could* do that—though he'd just go to a friend's house." "Perhaps, but even so you'd be giving him an important message, non-verbally, that home is a valuable place." "That's right."

It appeared that Mrs. Z was now getting with my moves toward less talk, less anxiety, and less defensiveness, and more effective—even if unusual— action. But not completely, as she went on to ask "But what about the day-time?" "Well, we have to take things one step at a time. But in general, I think when you want him to do something, you would be further ahead to say simply 'I'd like you to do such-and-such. But I can't make you do it. If you don't, I don't know what I'll do about it'." Mrs. Z really encouraged me by the way she picked upon this: "That might be good with Jacky; if he knows what's coming he can handle or evade it." However, I continued to take a doubting position, saying "Yes, but my bet is you won't be able to really do it. Jacky knows how to push your buttons—especially your guilt button—and get you involved in explaining to him. So you say you'll get with it, but I'll be ready to say 'I told you so' when you don't do it."

We set up another appointment, but just before that time Mrs. Z called to say she had car trouble and couldn't make it. However, she reported trying some things I'd suggested—mainly avoiding getting embroiled in arguments with Jacky—with positive results. But it had not been an easy week. "I certainly did not suggest or expect it would be easy. In fact, though I'm glad to hear you made some progress, I'm mostly surprised I don't get to point my 'I told you so' finger at you. But it's not easy to keep it up, so let's meet next week, and maybe I'll be able to point the finger then."

When she came in a week later, I immediately said "Do I get to point the finger at you?" (It would have been better to have said "I'm sure that now I get to point the finger.") She replied "No—he's been really good. Of course, I've backed off, not nagging so much (she had never recognized her talk as nagging before this)—though not perfect of course." In addition, she reported, though Jacky was still difficult in some ways, he was doing the jobs around the house willingly, and had voluntarily owned up to some matter involving taking money without asking: "He's so good I'm nervous, wondering what will happen next." "I expect probably the next little thing he does, you'll slip and blow it all." "Well, if I can just keep my temper—he really likes to get my goat."

Again I felt she was making considerable change and progress, so I moved to consolidate this, not by reassuring her but by asking "What might be the real acid test of his getting to you?" She said this would be if he went out and didn't come home, or even call—but went on to indicate that maybe she had already passed this test: She reported that he had stayed out late one night, and she had locked him out as suggested. When he did get home and she finally let him in, Jacky revealed that he had encountered a "weirdo" on the dark street and been scared; he was plainly glad to be home and safe. "Well, all right, you've handled that, but what about his smoking pot? " "I've backed off on talking about that—and Jacky has told me he only smokes it once a week now; when he's busy, he doesn't need it."

By this point, Mrs. Z was indicating positive changes and increasing confidence, loud and clear, and I was thinking about terminating treatment at the end of the session—since in my view she had made a basic change in her interaction with Jacky, and this should lead to further positive developments without continuing therapeutic intervention. However, in the time remaining, rather than shifting to a stance of optimism and congratulation, which might set her up for a discouraging let-down as soon as she encountered any difficult situation—which inevitably would occur—I kept on the same track of pointing out that she would meet further difficulties, but there were ways by which she might handle them. I suggested that, especially since Mr. Z had really gotten involved in the therapy, some problems between him and Jacky, and also Mr. Z and herself, probably would still arise. She agreed. I proposed that she could help improve the relationship between father and son by telling Jacky that she knew from much personal experience that his father was a difficult man, rather than defending him, or otherwise indicating that Jacky really should get together readily with his father. Several ideas underlay this apparently negative recommendation: 1. Most important, previous efforts at encouraging them had not worked. 2. Such a change gets her out of the middle and out of an undue responsibility for their relationship. 3. It moves her toward a realistically equal or one-up position vis-a-vis her ex-husband via justifiable criticism of him, and thus away from her previous guilty and one-down status. 4. It presents Jacky with a realistic challenge, to which he is likely to respond better than to "Why don't you get along better with your father?" which implies that this is no difficult matter, and therefore he is an incompetent failure if the relationship does not go well, easily and at once.

As to Mrs. Z's own relationship with her ex-husband, I suggested that if and when Mr. Z should again get on her case, especially by stating or implying that Jacky's problems were her fault, she could really blow him out of the water just by verbally agreeing with his accusations. My underlying idea here was that with Mr. Z, as with Jacky, Mrs. Z had been stuck in a position of overt defensive argument which only fed and prolonged her underlying feelings of guilt; verbal agreement would cut the argument short, while her own reaction to making such an overt statement would be "Really, it's not all my fault."

And finally, I suggested, when Jacky returned to school and met difficulties there, as he inevitably would, she could help him best not by direct encouragement, but by saying "I expect you to work at your studies, but even when you do, after all the mess-up you've been in before, I'm not at all sure you can hack it." Again, my aim was to get her to stop an approach which had been getting nowhere, and to substitute a challenge to which Jacky might respond—if only (but in a way that would require constructive efforts) to prove her wrong. I then dismissed her with the message—still maintaining my doubting or pessimistic stance—that of course she'd have more tests to face with Jacky; I was not sure whether she'd pass them or not, but she knew where to call me if she did not.

I did not receive any further calls. Seven months later I called her and asked how things were going. She said that while there were some ups and downs, generally things were much better; it seems it was right to bring Jacky back to live with her. To this I agreed. She also mentioned that she recalls some of the things I told her, and uses them at times, though "I may feel I have a bleeding tongue"—that is, she has to bite back some of her old reactions. I agreed that it is often an effort to do the right thing, she thanked me for calling, and I hung up feeling that some significant change had been initiated in our assorted phone calls and four actual sessions.

## References

Weakland, J., Fisch, R, Watzlawick, P. & Bodin, A. (1974). "Brief Therapy: Focused Problem Resolution," *Family Process*, 13 141-168.

Watzlawick, P., Weakland, J., & Fisch, R. (1974). *Change: Principles of Problem Formation & Problem Resolution.* New York, Norton.

Maruyama, M. (1963). "The Second Cybernetics: Deviation-Amplifying Mutual Causative Processes", *American Scientist*, 51, 164-I 79.

Wender, P.H. (1968). "Vicious & Virtuous Circles: The Role of Deviation Amplifying Feedback in the Origin and Perpetuation of Behavior", *Psychiatry*, *31,* 309-324.

# CHAPTER 10

# Pursuing the Evident
# Into Schizophrenia and Beyond[1]

## *John H. Weakland*

When "Toward a Theory of Schizophrenia" (Bateson, Jackson, Haley, & Weakland, 1956) was published, the double bind idea it set forth was something very new—yet it can now be seen that in some very basic respects this concept was only pursuing what was already evident. This concept made a breakthrough whose applications and consequences have been sizable and widespread—yet what has developed from it in the past 20 years appears quite limited.

These statements seem contradictory, and they are, but not insolubly. The contradictions rest upon the unlabeled use of different levels of reference for the term "double bind." Viewed broadly, this practice is nothing new, and it has been a source of considerable confusion and controversy over most of the brief history of the double bind concept. Our original article described a pattern of communication we labeled the double bind and its presumed relationship to schizophrenia at a rather general level of specification. Our follow-up attempts at further clarification and specification (Bateson, Jackson, Haley, & Weakland, 1963; Weakland, 1960) were pitched at a similar level. Much of the subsequent comment, criticism and inquiry about the double bind has aimed at

[1] Reprinted from *Beyond the double bind: Communication & family systems, Theories, & techniques with schizophrenics,* M. Berger (Ed.), (1978), New York, Brunner/Mazel, pp. 85-96.

description or testing at a more detailed and specific level. As I have indicated elsewhere (Weakland, 1974), I think this direction of approach has largely missed the point, seeking precision of detail at the cost of losing track of the main ideas (Cf. also Bateson, et. al., 1956). In any event, my aim here is very different: by reviewing the double bind concept even more broadly than in the original presentation—and within the broadest relevant context—to shed some new light on the nature and significance of this idea, while resolving the contradictions with which I began.

What was and is the double bind concept, anyway? It appears by now to have been many things to many people, perhaps almost as many as the number of those who have written about or discussed it. It also appears to have been nothing to far more—that is, all those to whose work and thinking it could be relevant and useful, but who have paid it only passing attention, *or* none. Still, avoiding any attempt to define the double bind completely, or claim to state its essence one thing may safely be said: At the very beginning the double bind concept represented  an attempt to understand certain phenomena of human life—those classified as "schizophrenia"—by relating them to a pattern of communication identified by describing its basic interrelated elements, and labeled as the "double bind." How well this aim was realized is, for the moment, beside the point.

Throughout the study of communication and behavior there is emphasis on the importance of understanding things in context, so it seems only appropriate to consider our own endeavor in context. Again, there is no claim to comprehensiveness—there are many contexts of any behavior—but one relevant and important context is plain enough. The double bind formulation was one example of the broad class of attempts to explain human events and situations.

## Explanatory Schema

In all times and places, apparently, people have not just lived; they have also sought to explain (and using such explanations, to better predict and control) life situations of importance to them. "Situations of importance" especially includes strange and difficult ones, for these obviously pose problems of understanding and control. There may be satisfaction in explaining the ordinary, or even the exceptionally good, but there is no necessity in it. Since what we can know and understand by direct perception or intuition is limited at best, and communication of any such understanding even more so, such explanation necessarily involves interpretation and conceptualization—the construction of mental, which means largely verbal, maps of the world of human events (Watzlawick, 1976).

The potential number of explanatory systems probably is infinite, and certainly there is an enormous variety actually existing and observable. Yet at a very general level, three main lines of interpretation can be distinguished. First, there is what could be termed the impersonal causation view. In this view, human events and problems are seen as consequences of large and powerful forces external to the realm of human behavior. If behavior is involved at all, it is only as a result of such forces, or in struggling with them; the prime mover is elsewhere. These forces may be supernatural—fate, demons, or the will of God. They may be forces of physical nature—the influence of climate or geography. They may even be social, but in so broad a sense as to be impersonal—the economic, political, or technological system. In modern times particularly, the list has been extended to include small but powerful forces—microbes, genes and drugs.

Second, there is the personal causation view. In this view events and, most especially, problems are seen as consequences of inherent personal characteristics attributed to some individual or to some group of individuals. These characteristics may be mental—inferior intelligence or irrationality; moral—greed, sloth or lust; or physical—bodily handicap or constitutional type. Some kind of bad or mad behavior may be seen as constituting the immediate problem, but this behavior is just the surface manifestation of the inner personal characteristic. Typically, "They are making trouble (for us), because they are aggressive."

There are also, of course, overlaps or combinations of these two views, as in theories of climate and racial character, but these need no special attention here. What matters more is that such general interpretive view—whether or not these are "true" or "appropriate" in any given instance, if indeed this can ever be determined with certainty—have correspondingly broad implications and consequences of great significance for understanding and dealing with human problems. Moreover, although the "impersonal" and the "personal" interpretive viewpoints appear to be polar opposites, their implications often are quite similar.

First, as to the *nature* of problems, from both viewpoints problems tend to be seen as external and isolated, at least relative—that is, as an event or an action "out there" which happens to or impinges on someone. In addition, the nature of any problem is generally seen as simple and self-evident. There may be a question of why it exists, but hardly any of *what* a given problem is.

Ideas about *causation* of problems closely parallel such ideas about their nature. If problems are viewed as external, so naturally are their causes; something out there leads to the particular event in nature, or act of someone, that constitutes a problem for the person whose life is impinged upon. Also, as problems are seen in rather isolated and concrete terms, so too with causation. At the extreme—but a common extreme—this leads to seeking for *the* cause of any problem. Further, though it is not really inherent in either the impersonal or personal viewpoint, their common tendency to see events and especially difficulties as discrete entities and as "outside" the subject leads readily to a linear concept of causation and its associated emphasis on origins—"Event Y happened to me, with Z as its result. So what was the X that led to Y?" and so on back.

It may be noted that all of the foregoing is based, implicitly, on observation and interpretation from the subject's viewpoint—that of the person or persons encountering the problem. Yet this, after all, is everyone's natural starting point. We are all self-centered, first and foremost, and even when we aim to consider events as more detached observers, we still must do so through our own eyes and minds. Indeed, one curious apparent exception to this, and one very relevant to our own special field of interest, at bottom turns out to be more of the same. Some problems are seen as arising from causes within the subject rather than without. Yet, typically, even here the conception, on either an impersonal or personal view, is "The cause is *in* me, but not *of* me." In another terminology, it is labeled as "ego-alien." "I am possessed by evil spirits; my disease is caused by invading microbes; my behavior results in difficulties (for myself or for another), but it is involuntary, or someone is making me act so; *I* am not really doing it." Once again, the view is that something essentially separate and distinct, even if now inside, is impacting on the subject to cause a problem.

Finally, these views carry implications about dealing with or *handling* problems. Corresponding to ideas of *the* cause, there are searches for *the* solution. Since problems are seen as external in basic nature—most involve the impact of external factors on the subject—solutions must be directed outward; either impersonal forces or other people must be changed to resolve a problem. And not least, though particular solutions envisioned to different problems may vary, there is a strong tendency toward extremism—either that nothing can be done, or that only major efforts and major change will be of any use. Such extremism follows rather naturally from the ideas that the source of trouble is external to oneself, so not within easy reach, and is powerful and hard to influence because it is impersonal, or perhaps worse, personal in an inherently bad way. But such views lead, all too readily, to massive and costly efforts at final solutions. It may be wondered whether, in general, it is worse when these fail or when they succeed.

Of course, no single explanatory scheme will suit best for everything, and there certainly are human difficulties and problems for which one of these two views may be most appropriate in guiding understanding and action. Concrete and practical difficulties immediately resulting from natural disasters, accidents, or unprovoked violence come readily to mind. But the kind of problems people bring to psychotherapists typically are different from these. While clinical problems may sometimes appear as arising out of or related to specific concrete difficulties, more often no striking or dramatic origin is evident, or a patient appears to read catastrophe into an ordinary difficulty of life. In any case, what appears characteristic of clinical problems is apparent helplessness—inaction or useless action—in the face of some constant or recurrent difficulty.

## The Interactional View

There is, however, a third general model of events and problems, a view quite different in nature and implications from both the impersonal and the personal views. Most broadly, this might be called the interactional view, or, with a narrower focus on human situations and behavior, the interpersonal view. Basically, this view relates what is occurring—regardless of whether this is labeled as good or bad, a desirable state of affairs or a problem to be resolved—to interaction within some system of ongoing interrelationships. In such a view, problems and their causes are not "out there," as isolated external factors; they are right here, as part of the system—which for clinical problems consists of the identified patient and other significant members of his social system, especially the family. Since such systems may be complex and have not been much examined, even for obvious "problems," the nature of the situation—the *what* of the problem—should not be taken as self-evident. Instead, in the interactional view, the first matter of inquiry is *what* is happening; and the next, rather than *why*, is *how* is this happening. That is, how does the overall system of interaction fit together, function and maintain itself, and how does any part specifically focused on fit into the context of the system? But this leads to a very different view of causation—not a linear view with one thing leading to another and to still another over time, but a cybernetic view whose focus is on circularity and feed-back causal loops, and on how these serve to maintain (or alter) the going system, rather than on its origins.

The implications of this view for the handling of problems are also very different. For instance, the very notion of a system implies that all its "parts" are interconnected (though not that all parts and relationships are necessarily of equal importance). In clinical problems, this means that the patient and any significant others are in it—the problem—together. Accordingly, resolution of a problem requires change in the system of interaction—but equally, a change initiated at any point in the system provokes change throughout it. Moreover, such a view plainly puts more emphasis on the observable here and now of interaction, as well as on potential alterations of this system, than on the past. Still other implications of this interactional viewpoint, to be mentioned later, have become clear only in recent years.

For some time now, the interactional explanatory view has been growing more important in a variety of areas. This, for instance, is the essential basis of ecological thinking. What seems curious is that its application directly to human behavior and problems has been limited, although it is precisely there that this viewpoint appears rather a simple and evident one, whose relevance is open to direct observation, and a familiar everyday matter. All of us may incline toward personal (or sometimes impersonal) explanations for matters in which we are immediately and closely involved—at least there is a certain comfort in seeing problems as "out there." But everyone also has had opportunities to note that how one person deals with another, by actions and by words, may influence that other strongly, and at many levels—his thinking, feeling, speaking, and other behavior—and that how the other responds in turn similarly influences the first, and so on indefinitely in any ongoing relationship.

To cite a more specific but common example, even a layman may see that in a marital conflict between two people he knows, both husband and wife are saying and doing things—in "self-defense," or all too often even in well-meant but inappropriate attempts to help the situation—that provoke the other and serve to maintain the conflict. It may be quite apparent to the observer that if either of the two parties would only take a different line of approach with the spouse, the conflict might cool down and end. In short, especially in the field of human behavior and relationships, the interactional view is old, common, and evident.

## Interaction and Schizophrenia

It is equally evident, though, that this view is apt to be ignored or overlooked, and the impersonal or personal model used when the going gets rough. As suggested, the going is always rougher when one is personally involved. Beyond that, however, the interactional view is rather regularly left aside—or at most, used in a minimal, limited way—when extreme or unusual events or actions are the focus of attention; that is, precisely where problems are concerned, and the more so the more these are seen as serious ones. Although the idea is not usually made quite explicit, it is as if, where either very destructive ("bad") or very odd ("mad") behavior is in question, everyone takes the stance "That behavior is just too much to account for by the influence of human interaction," or "Even if that looks like behavior, it is really not behavior—it is some other kind of action, caused by demons, or by his illness," or whatever.

Schizophrenia, of course, is a prime example of extreme behavior, very odd in a variety of bewildering ways, and often enough destructive too. Accordingly, it has most commonly and traditionally not been seen as behavior at all in the ordinary sense, but as speech and action beyond the pale. Schizophrenics observably act and speak, but "irrational actions" and "word-salad" were not classified as behavior but as "craziness," a different category. Correspondingly, special causal explanations have been sought for such words and actions, and for the state of schizophrenia they are presumed to exemplify. Those proposed have been many and varied, covering the gamut from impersonal (physiological dysfunction) through mixed (genetic factors), to personal (some profound trauma imposed on the helpless infant).

Against this context—and with the aid of hindsight—our original work on schizophrenia and the double bind can be seen as an attempt to examine schizophrenia, deliberately and persistently, in terms of the interactional explanatory model: to relabel schizophrenia as behavior, and to look at its environing context of communication and interaction to see just where and how far pursuing this viewpoint might lead.

At least after it once got under way this pursuit was, as stated, deliberate and persistent. That is not to claim that it was clear, simple, and direct. We made progress, but it was gradual, sometimes halting, with false steps and sidetracks. The original double bind paper, for instance referred considerably to "binders" and "victims." In doing so, despite our general emphasis on communicative interaction, it leaned toward a personal explanatory view, pinning the causal blame mostly on the "schizophrenogenic mother" as villain. Also, in this and in speaking as if there were no possible positive responses to the double bind pattern—only a choice among crazy ones, linear causation was implicit, despite our broader emphasis on cybernetic ideas of causation. Even though we soon made attempts at explanation, modification and correction (Bateson, et. al, 1963; Weakland, 1960), these ideas did exist in our original article, and their ghosts still remain to haunt us and the whole field. Yet I think it is fair to claim that our main thrust was toward stating and applying an interactional view; this is the meaning of my statement that our "new" work consisted of pursuing the evident into schizophrenia, a formerly segregated domain.

## Beyond Schizophrenia

What, then, does the "beyond" of my title refer to? First, in the 20 years since "Towards a Theory of Schizophrenia" was published, the interactional view has progressively become more widely applied to problems of understanding and action, while also being clarified and made more explicit.

Almost as soon as schizophrenia had been discussed in terms of communication and interaction, this viewpoint began to be extended to other problems of "mental illness" and deviant behavior, until—in a relatively short time—

most of the clinical problems commonly met in psychotherapy were being considered anew in this light (cf. Sluzki & Vernon, 1971). It was as if a door had been opened; if this approach was useful in understanding the very serious and protean syndrome of schizophrenia, what might it not accomplish elsewhere, in simpler and more limited problems?

Meanwhile, developments in practice paralleled those in research and explanatory description. With schizophrenia itself, direct observation and study of how patients and their family members interacted communicatively led very rapidly to attempts to alter their interaction for the better—that is, to treatment. Moreover, the spread from an initial focus on schizophrenia to concern with the whole spectrum of common clinical problems took place there too, with practice just as with observation and inquiry. The double bind view of schizophrenia thus was one of the primary sources of the development of family therapy in general, though of course not the only one.

Another broader development has been the continuing and increasing attention given to the general nature of communication, and its significance. The double bind concept itself followed, and probably depended upon, earlier insights in the Bateson group about the particular importance of complexity and multiplicity in all communication, and especially human communication—the pervasive existence of multiple channels and levels of messages, mutually qualifying or framing one another. Since then there has been increasing spread of these ideas about communication and its importance in structuring and maintaining both problems and normal social behavior (Watzlawick, Beavin-Bavelas, & Jackson, 1967). There have been costs consequent on this increased awareness of the significance of communication—the term has become a cliche and a pseudo-explanation, as in "Our problem is that we don't communicate"—but perhaps the gains outweigh the cost. There has been rather less development of new insights, with two exceptions. It is probably clearer now than before that the enormous influence and power of communication do not derive just from the fact that it taps into or activates the energy sources within a human system. This power also depends on the fact that not only does all communication involve interpretation, but human living itself is basically a matter of interpretation—"There is nothing either good or bad, but thinking makes it so"—guided by communication (Watzlawick, 1976). And since one message can confirm or reframe (that is, guide the interpretation of) another message or a whole series of other messages, communication always involves a sort of multiplicative or exponential power.

Finally, and most important, the epistemological view inherent in our work on schizophrenia and the family, as well as its implications, has been clarified, spread, and utilized. It has already been suggested that our original study involved a basic shift from a linear concept of causation to a cybernetic model concerned primarily with current interaction among the elements of a system. In "Cybernetic Explanation," Bateson (1967) has expanded on the general nature and significance of this view. The range of human situations considered in terms of this viewpoint has gradually but significantly expanded (Watzlawick & Weakland, 1977). And gradually, its profound implications concerning the origin, maintenance, and effective handling of clinical problems are becoming clearer. Most fundamentally, from this viewpoint, problems are no longer a quantitative matter. Instead, interactionally, both problem formation and problem resolution are organizational matters. Accordingly, there is no necessary similarity between the size or severity of a problem (which is always a matter of human evaluation anyway) and either the original or precipitating cause or the action needed to resolve it. Therefore, there is no extremist implication of "Either give up and suffer the problem, or mount an attack of great enough power and duration to lick it." Rather, in a system of interaction, because there are feedback loops and energy sources within the system, a small change provoked from without may be strategic in reorganizing interaction, leading to progressive further change by taking advantage of the workings of the system itself (Maruyama, 1963; Watzlawick, Weakland, & Fisch, 1974; Weakland, 1977; Weakland, Fisch, Watzlawick, & Bodin, 1974). In simplest terms, by actions more concerned with conveying new information than applying effort or power, a beneficent circle may be instituted, and resolved problems disappear rather than being overcome.

## Beyond the Present

Yet all this, from another perspective, appears not so much. Even among those interested in this viewpoint, both its explanatory and practical applications have been limited. For instance, while the interactional view has been rather widely used in the understanding and treatment of "mad" behavior—that is, various sorts of "mental illness"—much less has been done concerning "bad" behavior—problems involving violence or other uncontrolled action. A beginning has undeniably been made, especially with problems of "uncontrollable" children and juvenile delinquency. But this is only a beginning. The term still commonly applied to such problems, "acting-out," itself carries implications of a limited scope of interest, as well as the suggestion that something underlying, an inner causal factor, should be the focus of attention. Not much has been done from an interactional viewpoint to examine or treat really violent behavior, even on the clinical scale—such as child abuse—and almost nothing on the wider social scale, despite the obvious importance of violent behavior in today's world.

Clinically, also, the interactional view has until now largely been concerned with, and restricted to, "mental" or "emotional" problems. The one significant exception only makes clearer what so far is scanted. There has been significant family-oriented work on a few common psychosomatic problems, particularly by Minuchin and his co-workers (1975) and by Selvini-Palazzoli's group in Milan (1970). Even this work has largely been limited to problems where an emotional factor is rather plain, as with asthma, or where the family's management of an illness is evidently a crucial matter, as with diabetes and anorexia nervosa. Many other psychosomatic problem have as yet received no significant attention from this perspective. And beyond all that, there is the whole untouched area of real disease—problems now ordinarily conceived as basically, or completely, organic in nature. At the very least, the management and course of many organic diseases may be significantly influenced, for good or ill, by the kind of interaction between the patient and the family members—or patient and physician. Hoebel's exploration of spousal influence on high-risk behaviors among coronary artery patients (Hoebel, 1977) is one case in point. But we also know that physiological functioning certainly can be altered temporarily by communicative means. Threats, disastrous news, glad tidings and many other kinds of messages can all have observable bodily effects, not to mention the more extensive and profound effects producible by that special form of communicative interaction called hypnosis. What we do not know—some recent work on cancer is a start in this direction, but only that—is how much effect on organic functioning persistent patterns of interaction may have, and this would be worth finding out (Weakland, 1977).

What has been done so far has also been limited in another way. The interactional view has been largely applied to only one system, that of the family. There are partial exceptions to this, it is true. Bateson has examined a variety of problems, especially some in biology and evolution, from a cybernetic viewpoint (Bateson, 1972). And closer to hand, in relation to children's school problems, there is some movement among clinicians toward viewing the school as well as the family as a system of interaction. But the world is full of ongoing organizations—business, labor, social, governmental and others—that relate to problems important in people's lives. Even allowing for certain work in anthropology, sociology, and political science, it appears that not very much has been done to apply the interactional view seriously to this wider area of social systems beyond the family. If we did, perhaps ultimately we might even understand "the family of nations" more adequately than we do now.

All this, of course, only represents hopeful thinking. As Murray Bowen pointed out so well in this conference itself, at present the family or interactional view, in any form or degree, is distinctively a minority one even within our own immediate fields of psychiatry and psychology.

The broad future of the interactional viewpoint is correspondingly uncertain. The only thing we may be sure of is that there is much left to pursue.

## References

Bateson, G. (1966). Slippery theories, *International Journal of Psychiatry*, 2, 415-417.

Bateson, G. (1967). Cybernetic explanation. *American Behavioral Scientist*,10 (8), 29-32.

Bateson, G. (1972). *Steps to an Ecology of Mind,* New York: Ballantine Books.

Bateson, G., Jackson, D., Haley, J., & Weakland, J. (1956). Toward a theory of schizophrenia. *Behavioral Science*, 1 (1), 251-264.

Bateson, G., Jackson, D., Haley, J., & Weakland, J. (1963). A note on the double bind-1962. *Family Process*, 2, 154.161.

Hoebel, F. (1977). Coronary artery disease and family interaction: A study of risk factor modification. In: P. Watzlawick & J. Weakland (Eds.), *The Interactional View*. New York: Norton, 1977.

Maruyama, M. (1963). The second cybernetics: Deviation amplifying mutual causal processes. In: W. Buckley (Ed.), (1963). *Modern Systems Research for the Behavioral Scientist*. Chicago: Aldine.

Minuchin, S., Baker, L., Rosman, B., Libman, R., Milman, L., & Todd, T. (1975). A conceptual model for psychosomatic illness in children: Family organization & family therapy. *Archives of General Psychiatry*, 32, 1031-1038.

Selvini-Palazzoli, M. (1970). The families of patients with anorexia nervosa. In: E. Anthony & C. Koupernik (Eds.),(1970). *The Child in His Family*. New York: Wiley.

Sluzki, C., & Vernon, E. (1971). The double bind as a universal pathogenic situation. *Family Process*, 10, 397-410.

Watzlawick, P. (1976). *How Real Is Real?* New York: Random House.

Watzlawick, P., Beavin, J. , & Jackson, D. (1967). *Pragmatics of Human Communication*. New York: Norton.

Watzlawick, P., Weakland, J. & Fisch, R. (1974). *Change: Principles of Problem Formation and Problem Resolution*. New York: Norton, 1974.

Watzlawick, P. & Weakland, J. (Eds.).(1977). The Interactional View: Studies at the Mental Research Institute, Palo Alto, 1965-1974. New York: Norton, 1977.

Weakland, J. (1960). The "double-bind" hypothesis of schizophrenia & three-party interaction. In: D. Jackson (Ed.), *The Etiology of Schizophrenia*. New York: Basic.

Weakland, J. (1974). "The double bind theory" by self-reflexive hindsight.

*Family Process*, 13, 269-277.

Weakland, J. (1977). "Family somatics"—A neglected edge. In: P. Watzlawick & J. Weakland (Eds.), *The Interactional View.* New York: Norton.

Weakland, J., Fisch, R., Watzlawick, P., & Bodin, A. (1974). Brief therapy: Focused problem resolution. *Family Process*, 13, 141-168.

Wender, P.(1968). Vicious & virtuous circles: The role of deviation amplifying feedback in the origin & perpetuation of behavior. *Psychiatry*, 31, 309-324.

# CHAPTER 11

# The Double-Bind Theory: Some Current Implications for Child Psychiatry[1]

## John H. Weakland

*The behavioral-interactional view of problems in the original statement of the double bind theory is outlined and the broad significance of this viewpoint for treatment is discussed. Recent emphasis on the cybernetic causal model is noted, and its implications for family therapy in general and for child-centered problems in particular are reviewed. A case example of brief treatment of hyperactivity based on this approach is described.*

The double-bind theory, originally set forth by Bateson, Jackson, Haley, and Weakland (1956), together with contemporary work on the family and schizophrenia and on families with very difficult adolescents constitute the main bases from which family therapy arose (Guerin, 1976). The concepts described by Bateson et al. embody most of the ideas concerning problems, families, and interaction that are still central to the theory and practice of the communications school of family therapy today, including family treatment of problems involving children primarily. It therefore seems worth reviewing the

---

[1] Originally published in the *Journal of the American Academy of Child Psychiatry*, (1979), 18, 54-66.

main premises and concepts involved in the double-bind theory for understanding the treatment of child-centered problems. This consideration of the implications and effects of the double-bind theory will focus initially and largely on its general features. The original double-bind theory was not a stopping point, but a starting point, for theory and practice. Weakland (1974) noted that the concepts were fundamentally concerned with the general relationship between behavior and communication, and with an approach to investigating the nature and significance of this relationship. It is the development and application of this orientation that appears as increasingly important to psychiatry in general—here defined broadly as the understanding and treatment of problems of human behavior—and child psychiatry in particular.

What are the basic elements of this view of communication and behavior? First, that the "problems" with which therapists generally deal consist primarily of *behavior* and should be considered as such—even when the behavior involved is as extreme or extraordinary as occurs in schizophrenia or some kinds of interpersonal violence (Weakland, 1978). Second, that a most important aspect of social (non-isolated) behavior lies in its communicative effects, while equally communication is a major factor in the ordering of behavior (including both action and verbal behavior) socially. In contrast to other views which consider behavior to be an external manifestation of individual characteristics, innate or learned early in life, the communicational view proposes that behavior depends mainly on *maintenance* of patterns by repeated reinforcement in social interaction in the ongoing here and now. Third, communication is basically and pervasively interactive and systematic. While people often make unidirectional *attributions* of messages and effects ("I withdraw because she nags me"), in any ongoing relationship behavioral influence is circular (the other half of the circle of interaction being "I nag because he withdraws"). Communicative interaction is systematic in the sense that messages and their effects do not occur at random in couples, in families, or in any ongoing social group. Rather, repetitive patterns develop, often rapidly, and these may become so persistent as to appear fixed—for example, to seem an expression of set personality traits of the individuals involved. Yet the possibility of change of behavior in response to altered communication always exists.

Such a view makes sense only if communication itself is considered or conceived in a way that has not been usual. Ordinarily, communication has been considered and studied as the transmission of information; from this an ideal of simplicity and clarity of communication naturally follows. The position basic to the double-bind theory, however, is very different. In this view, human communication is not simple but complex. Messages occur not in isolation but in the context of other related messages; ongoing exchange of messages largely constitutes what usually are termed relationships. The significance of any message singled out for attention can only be estimated in relation to its context, not by any form of analysis of the message itself. Furthermore, even an analytically isolated single message is complex, involving multiple channels of communication—words, tone, facial expression and so on. The import of these different channels may be similar or congruent and therefore mutually reinforcing. But the import of these channels may also be different and incongruent either grossly or subtly (as "Yes" can, according to how it is said, convey anything from "Certainly" to "Not really").

Moreover, Bateson et al. proposed that every message conveys both a report (information) and a command (influence). It is this influential aspect of communication that is most significant in determining behavior for good or bad, persistence or change. Information itself, in the common but restricted sense of "facts," is influential, but there is much more to it than this. Misinformation may be as influential as facts, conflicting messages may produce conflictful responses, and messages may influence general premises, including those determining the whole tone of interpersonal relationships, as well as specific ideas and actions.

Once we begin to consider communicative influence, it is possible to glimpse some cogent reasons why communication may affect behavior powerfully. In the first place, human behavior is based, not on direct perception of a response to reality, but on some *interpretation* of the natural and human environment—on conceptual maps, if you will—whether these are more or less explicit. Communication, especially verbal formulations about human events and relationships, is crucial in determining such interpretations. This holds equally whether a given message is such as to maintain (reinforce) an existing interpretation, or to alter it. Further, the effect of communication is multiplicative, in two ways. First, communication is not a physical force but a signal; it taps and directs the energy of the receiver. A new idea may be much more potent than a shout. Second, one brief message may serve to alter the interpretation of many other messages or behaviors, prospectively or even retrospectively (I admit that I did and said all that you charge me with, but it was involuntary, so I am not responsible"—i.e., I did it, but I didn't really *do* it.")

At the same time, while there are ample reasons to recognize the potential power of communication to shape and organize behavior, this does not tell us what particular kinds of communication, in what particular circumstances, lead to what effects, nor what the limits of communicative influence may be, nor how it may be used deliberately to alleviate problems. These are more specific and empirical questions, answerable only by experiment and experience. In my view, Bateson et al. posed such questions, and much of the subsequent development of family study and treatment is best understood as an exploration of them.

Just as the double-bind theory—or more generally, the interactional view of behavior—was based on a variety of conceptual and observational sources, so also it had a variety of implications. Obviously one of these was toward application in clinical practice. Once problems are seen as primarily matters of behavior, and behavior is seen as greatly influenced (if not primarily determined) by communication and interaction among the individuals composing a social system, it no longer seems reasonable to consider a patient in isolation, and his symptomatic behavior as primarily a manifestation of inner defects. Rather, the only reasonable step is to bring the identified patient together with the other members of his family (as the most basic social system) for study and treatment. Using direct observation in addition to verbal inquiry, such study correspondingly focuses on their current interaction, particularly on how the behavior of the other members may lead, even if unintentionally and unwittingly, to the disturbed behavior of the patient. Therapy similarly becomes focused on attempts to change such pathogenic patterns of interaction in order to improve the functioning both of the identified patient and of the family as a whole. In addition, such a focus on a need for change in family communication patterns, which involve complex, mutually reinforcing interaction, implies that the therapist must intervene as an active agent of change.

These views constituted the basic conceptual foundation for the first attempts to apply the double-bind theory by treating schizophrenics in the family context. Quite soon thereafter the family approach to treatment was expanded from this base and its other base, family work with certain child problems, toward application to the whole spectrum of recognized psychiatric problems, except the manifestly organic. This too was logical enough, since the viewpoint involved was fundamentally a general one, not specific to schizophrenia, and since schizophrenia is such a varied and extreme problem that almost any other appeared relatively easier to treat. Furthermore, once initiated, the practice of family therapy has grown greatly over the past 20 years. Nevertheless, these few and rather simple ideas still appear as basic to the practice of family therapy generally. They also are basic to a fundamental tenet of many in the field—that family therapy is not just an additional treatment technique, but involves a whole new conceptualization of problems and their resolution from which a new approach to practice derives.

Some of the orientations that developed in family therapy may be seen as involving a failure to pursue the fundamental premises fully. For example, there have been considerable tendencies, first evident in the original statement by Bateson et al. and persisting in spite of later corrective statements (e.g., Bateson et al., 1963) to view the identified patient as a sort of passive victim of conflicts or deficiencies elsewhere in the family. Young patients especially tended to be seen as overtly manifesting problems that really were centered in their parents' relationship. This notion seems more an inversion of prior views that stigmatized the patient as sick or bad than the broader and more balanced view that an interactional orientation calls for. As another example, some family therapists have become extensively involved (often with the family's help) in inquiry about the past history of the family or of the problem. While this might provide some information useful for understanding the present situation, more strictly it represents a digression from what the theory posed as central.

On another side, several tendencies developed in family therapy that may best be seen as deriving from eager but overspecific or literal reading of the basic principles, resulting in losing sight of more general and basic implications, and arriving at narrowed or distorted rules for practice. First, the idea of the family system and family influence led to prescriptions (e.g., Jackson and Weakland, 1961) that the entire family must always be seen in therapy, or even to expansion of the therapy group into "network therapy"' including grandparents, collaterals, and perhaps close neighbors (Speck and Attneave, 1971). Again seeing the whole family may have helped as a means of information gathering and understanding of interaction, especially in early family work when relationships between interaction and specific problems were hard to perceive, but the systems orientation does not imply this is essential for treatment, as will be discussed further on. Also, the concept of the family as a unitary system was at times taken to mean that the resolution of any problem must require a revision or restructuring of the whole family system, and the more severe the problem the wider and deeper this restructuring would need to be. This again is not an essential consequence of the interactional view. Further, the idea of the family as a system was closely associated with the concept of family homeostasis (Jackson, 1957); specific observations that patient improvement was often accompanied by new difficulties elsewhere in the family led to views that this *necessarily* would occur unless family therapy was rather deep and extensive instead of focused mainly around the presenting complaint—a family analogue of the concept of "symptom substitution" in individual therapy. An analogue to the concept of "insight" in individual treatment also developed, apparently related to recognition of the importance and power of communication. It is as if some family therapists became *too* aware of how problems could relate closely to vague or incongruent messages, and of the therapists own needs to see the nature of communicative interaction clearly and explicitly. At any rate, some therapists became almost exclusively involved in promoting "good"—simple, clear, and direct—communication to their patient families, usually by rather didactic analysis and instruction. Such practice neglected the fact that much normal human communication, not just the pathological, is complex or even contradictory, and that clear observation of what is going on may be very different from effective action to alter this.

Although it was recognized early that the double-bind viewpoint involves a cybernetic or circular model of causality rather than a linear one, the conceptual and practical implications of this have seldom been pursued fully. In this epistemological view, the behavior of any part ("individual") of a system ("family") is governed and is to be understood by reference to present organization and functioning of the system, not by past history. Applied to human problems this most fundamentally means that what is most significant is not why or even how a problem began, but how the problem behavior persists, which can occur only by repetitive performance. Basically, this is a positive feedback or vicious-circle view of problems (Maruyama, 1963; Wender, 1968). In this view the main focus of inquiry and intervention is that behavior by the patient and/or concerned others which—regardless of intentions—acts to maintain or escalate the problem behavior. Such a view also implies that there need be no similarity in size or nature between a current problem and its sources. A major problem may arise from an ordinary life difficulty, if this is persistently dealt with in a way that reinforces the difficulty rather than resolving it. Unfortunately, it appears that this may happen quite readily; for understandable reasons, people often get rigidly committed to inappropriate means of handling difficulties.

This cybernetic view of the nature of problems has powerful implications for all the major aspects of practice. First, if most problems are seen to consist of behavior, then it is important to focus inquiry and treatment as completely as possible on actual behavior: what people concretely do and say, here and now, rather than inner states or long-past events presumed to underlie observable behavior. Second, attention should be concentrated on the behavior constituting the problem and those behaviors most directly related to it (primarily people's behavior in dealing with the problem) rather than on family interaction in general. If it is necessary to look at behavior in the family, more widely, this will become evident, but it should not be assumed necessary in advance and in general. Third, if one takes the idea of systems quite seriously, its implication is not that the therapist must regularly see the whole family, but the reverse. If there is a system of interaction, while some change throughout the system may be necessary for resolution of a problem, potentially the entire system can be influenced through appropriate changes in any of its parts. Accordingly, so long as the interactional viewpoint is clearly kept in mind, whom to see in treatment becomes a question of strategic choice: who can best provide any necessary information, and who is most open to influence leading to useful change? Fourth, the basic task of the therapist becomes one of active intervention to interdict whatever behaviors are seen as functioning to maintain the problem behavior and to allow more appropriate behavior to occur instead, by whatever means are most effective in producing behavioral change. Fortunately, in this connection there is a very positive side to the cybernetic view of causation. It implies that, just as large problems may arise from small sources, even apparently complex and severe problems may not require heroic therapeutic measures and great changes for their resolution. An apparently small change, if it is strategic in effecting an alteration in the behavior maintaining the problem (rather than the problem behavior itself) may initiate a beneficent circle leading to further and progressive improvement.

The foregoing summarizes the concepts deriving from the double-bind view that we now see as most basic to family therapy, and their general implications for practice. Now let us consider their significance for the treatment of child-centered problems in particular: what sort of practice do such views lead to, and how is it different from traditional child psychiatric theory and practice.

## A Current Application of the Theory

The territory covered in a typical practice in child psychiatry is extensive and, on the surface, varied. Therefore, I will focus on describing the application of our typical approach to just one currently important child problem, contrasting this with the approach of traditional child psychiatry—which is admittedly my construct and somewhat of a straw man, set up only to help make clearer and more concrete the implications for practice of seriously pursuing the double-bind ideas, and how this differs from other approaches.

The problem selected is hyperactivity in children. In conceptualizing the nature of a problem which all else rests—traditional child psychiatry seldom sees the deviant behavior forming the presenting problem as both central to treatment and as behavior in the ordinary sense of the term. Instead the child's unusual or troublesome activities are often seen as involuntary, or as "only the tip of the iceberg," or both. The underlying and more significant matter (the "cause" or the "real" problem) is presumed to be located within the individual child patient. In nature this is commonly conceived as some kind of deficit, or at times the opposite, an excess of some factor. Rather curiously, in the case of hyperactivity, an apparent excess in behavior is often related to a presumed covert deficit, namely, "minimal brain damage." The "minimal brain damage" obviously refers to a presumed physiological deficit. Or the underlying factor may be conceived as belonging to the alternative class of causal factors, emotional in nature, e.g., anxiety. In this latter case, interpersonal influence may be deemed significant. However, major significance is attributed usually to early rather than current experience, and in any case the concerns about experience are likely to center around presumed emotional deprivations. Thus, this again is a deficit theory. Something is lacking in the constitution, or the experience, of the child and this makes him sick.

Correspondingly, treatment is focused largely on making up for such deficits, or at least compensating for them as much as possible, by therapeutic attempts in child problems generally to supply better understanding, more support, and perhaps reduced demands, plus special teaching or corrective drugs such as Ritalin for hyperactivity. In this view, too, the child is naturally seen as the primary object of treatment, though supplementary attention may be given to parents, largely directed toward helping them to understand and fulfill the child's needs better. This naturally is likely to involve special treatment of the child by the parents, in addition to that by teachers and therapist.

Finally, with this approach it may be somewhat difficult to evaluate improvement or resolution of the problem, since the child's behavior is often not itself seen as the fundamental matter, but rather as an indicator of something deeper and more covert. Observable changes in behavior can then hardly be an adequate criterion of progress, leaving one to rely on clinical judgment or psychological tests, both of which involve inference rather heavily.

The approach to hyperactivity deriving from the double-bind concept and its subsequent developments differs from the foregoing point by point. To begin with, superficial as it may seem, hyperactivity is viewed first and foremost as a problem of behavior, and handled and evaluated on this basis. The observable fact in hyperactivity, and indeed in many problems, is that a child is doing something that is judged (possibly by the child, but more usually by concerned others such as parents or teachers) as abnormally disturbing or harmful to the patient or others, and that this persists in spite of efforts to change it.

We would not be concerned about whether the problem was a matter of voluntary or involuntary behavior. This is a question which we believe is fundamentally insoluble and misleading (a more useful question would be: "Under what observable circumstances does such and such behavior occur, and under what circumstances does it not occur?"), although the views of the patient and others concerned with the problem about the voluntary or involuntary nature of the problem behavior are important to know.

Instead, in our practice, we would first aim to get a clear, concrete, and specific account of what behavior is seen as "hyperactive" and constituting a problem currently, *who* sees this behavior as a problem (the child patient may not), and *how* it is seen as constituting a problem. This is mainly done by direct, explicit, and if need be, persistent inquiry.

Our view thus sees the problem as consisting essentially—not just superficially—of concrete, identifiable, current behavior and related evaluations of such behavior as deviant. We avoid viewing behavior such as hyperactivity (or other common deviant child behaviors) as based on inner or experiential deficits unless there is plain and ample evidence for doing so, for two reasons.

First, failures to behave "normally" may occur readily as responses to situational factors (e.g., parent-child interaction), though these often will not be obvious; one must deliberately look for them. Second, even if some physiological or experiential deficit exists, the demands of everyday life really are not so great that passable performance is impossible despite deficits, if other factors are favorable—and we believe that improving the operating conditions of child and family constitutes the most hopeful and humane initial line of approach.

Since our viewpoint focuses on the maintenance of problems by other behavior within the family system as the central issue, we would next inquire, again specifically and concretely, about how the problem is being handled. We want to know what everyone concerned—including the patient, but with child problems especially the parents and involved others, if any seem significant—is doing and saying in their attempts to control, lessen, or alter the problem behavior. The reason for this is that we seek to identify the behavior that serves to maintain the problem—that unwittingly provokes or reinforces the problem behavior—as rapidly as possible. While theoretically this might be anything in the family's total behavioral repertoire, in practice this has quite regularly turned out to lie in the area of people's attempts to handle the problem. Correspondingly, the basic task of the therapist is not to support or compensate, but to identify what in the attempted "solutions" of the patient or family members is maintaining or exacerbating the problem behavior, despite their good intentions, and to change such behaviors as efficiently and expeditiously as possible.

This sort of approach obviously is likely to involve the parents as much as, or more than, the identified child patient. In fact, we often will see the child only once or twice, separately or with the parents, and thereafter see only them, with the aim of interdicting inappropriate handling of the child's behavior and replacing this with better ways. If such a change can be initiated, even a small first step may well start a beneficent circle of interaction going, even in severe problems. This allows the therapist to step aside soon, and let the cycle of social reinforcement of positive change within the family do the rest. Evaluation of the outcome of treatment, like evaluation of the original problem, is based on observation or report of concrete behavior.

Our goals in a case of hyperactivity would generally be toward reduction of the original hyperactive behavior (or, in some cases, reduction in parents' and others' evaluation of child behavior as indicating hyperactivity), return of the child to ordinary handling by parents and schools, and return of the parents to normal (less child-centered) social life.

Rather little has been said here about how therapists working on this basis intervene to promote such changes. A major part of the difficulty derives from the fact that such change involves getting parents (and sometimes others as well) to take actions with the hyperactive child very different from those they have been committed to, and often have seen as the only logical thing to do. Methods of promoting such change may vary considerably among different therapists and cases; they have been discussed elsewhere (Weakland et al., 1974; Watzlawick et al., 1974). Some general principles will now be mentioned, and one case example illustrating several means of promoting change will be summarized.

## A Clinical Example — The Use of Paradox as a Treatment Technique

With this approach, the basic goal is change of behavior, not insight or understanding of the problem—though these may follow successful change. The simplest method of promoting change is best if—but only if—it works. That is, if clients will follow direct requests or suggestions about handling a hyperactive child differently, fine. In our experience, though, this is rarely the case, although the odds may be improved somewhat by defining such a change as an experiment. Usually, however, to be effective suggestions for changes of behavior must be indirect. It is especially important to perceive the views and motivations that clients bring with them into therapy, and to reframe the problem situation in such a way that these motivations can lead to new and more useful behaviors—to offer an oversolicitous sacrificing mother the greater sacrifice of backing off, or the real challenge of making a change to a father who prides himself on capability—rather than trying to remake the individuals one is dealing with.

In hyperactivity as in other problems, sometimes the problem, in the sense of what needs to be changed, may lie not in the behavior of the child, but in the evaluation of this behavior. This, in essence, was the Brief Therapy Center's view of one particular case (Weakland and Fisch, 1976) in which the parents were "making a federal case" out of what appeared on specific and concrete inquiry to be rather ordinary misbehavior by their two sons, aged 12 and 13. Meanwhile, expectably, the boy's fanned the flames by exaggerated verbal accounts of their misdeeds, which the anxious and credulous parents received as gospel.

The parents' efforts to control the situation involved overkill treatment. This had proceeded from provocative futile warnings and nagging to attempts at 24-hour surveillance by the parents and school personnel in collusion. It had also included repeated medical examinations and diagnoses of hyperactivity resulting in medication first with Ritalin and then Thorazine. Finally, after a half-hour joyride in the family car, the younger son was incarcerated in Juvenile Hall for three months (the juvenile probation authorities were very reluctant about this, but the parents had been so anxious and insistent they felt forced to go along). At this point the family came to the Center.

This problem was resolved in 10 sessions, largely by pursuing three tactics. First, since the parents' anxiety was so obvious from their exaggerated accounts of the boys' "illness," we avoided any suggestion that they were making a mountain out of a molehill. Instead, paradoxically, we suggested they probably were minimizing the problem and giving us an overoptimistic view. At this, presumably feeling understood instead of opposed, they relaxed and backed off a bit. Second, the father was induced to take a firmer stand with the older son, who threatened aggressive behavior at times, by explanations that the boy needed reassurance that his father was strong enough to protect him if need be. Third, the mother was encouraged in her existing beliefs that she had certain powers of extrasensory communication with her sons, and given the suggestion that these could be used to control their behavior better than mere words could. This increased her confidence, decreased her anxiety, and helped her to stop her provocative verbal nagging and lecturing.

The family settled down, the boys began to get along at home and at school without further medication, and without need for further confrontation by father or ESP use by mother. A major sign of positive change, in our follow-up evaluation, was that the parents had begun to rebuild an active social life of their own, after half a dozen years of virtual "house arrest" for themselves, since they had not dared go out, leaving the boys without their direct surveillance, or invite friends in.

## Conclusion

In other cases, of course (as in the case of learning disability reported by Weakland, 1977), difficult child behaviors are more real and parental evaluation less exaggerated. Yet on the basis of the approach deriving from the double-bind theory that has been described here, the same principles apply in all child problems: identify the behavior that is serving to maintain the problem by inappropriate handling and, by reframing the situation to utilize the views and motives of the participants, help people to abandon their unhelpful "solutions" and try new ways of dealing with their children's behavior.

# References

Bateson, G., Jackson, D., Haley, J., & Weakland, D. (1956). Toward a theory of schizophrenia. *Behavioral Science* 1:251-264.

Bateson, G., Jackson, D., Haley, J., & Weakland, D (1963). A note on the double bind 1962. *Family Process*, 2:154-161.

Guerin, P., (1978). Family therapy. In: P. Guerin, (Ed.), *Family Therapy*, New York: Gardner Press. p. 2-22.

Jackson, D. (1957), The question of family homeostasis. *Psychiatric Quarterly*, 31(I): 79 -90.

Jackson, D., & Weakland, D. (1961). Conjoint family therapy. *Psychiatry.* 24. Supp. 2:30-45.

Maruyama, M (1963). The second cybernetics. *American Scientist,* 51:164-179.

Speck, R., & Attneave, C. (1971). Social network intervention. In: J. Haley (Ed.), *Changing Families*, New York: Grune & Stratton. p. 312-332.

Watzlawick, P., Weakland, J., & Fisch, R. (1974). *Change.* New York: Norton.

Weakland, J. (1974). Doublebind theory by self-reflexive hindsight. *Family Process*, 13: 269-277.

Weakland, J. (1978). Pursuing the evident into schizophrenia and beyond. In: M. Berger, (Ed.), *Beyond the Double Bind.* New York: Brunner/Mazel

Weakland, J. (1977). "OK-You've been a bad mother." In: P. Papp, (Ed.), *Family Therapy*, New York: Gardner Press, pp. 23-33.

Weakland, J., & Fisch, R. (1976), Brief therapy, in D. Ross & M. Ross (Eds.), *Hyperactivity*, New York: Wiley, pp. 176-182.

Weakland, J., Fisch, R., Watzlawick, P., & Bodin, A. (1974). Brief therapy, *Family Process*, 13:141-168.

Wender, P. (1968), Vicious & virtuous circles. *Psychiatry*, 31:317-324.

# CHAPTER 12

# "Family Therapy" with Individuals[1]

## John H. Weakland

## Summary

The interactional view that problem behavior occurs in the context of, and is maintained by, other behaviors, is seen as the basic premise of family therapy in general. It is proposed that not all environing behaviors are important. "Attempted solutions" are primary—and if these premises are taken seriously, it follows that it is not necessary to see whole families routinely. Advantages of seeing individual in certain kinds of situations are outlined. As a counterpoint, the application of the same interactional viewpoint to apparently "individual" problems is considered briefly.

My title, "'Family Therapy with Individuals" may seem obscure or self-contradictory to some, while to various others it may convey apparently clear but different meanings. I will therefore begin by stating as clearly and explicitly as I can what I propose to discuss here and, not less important, the basic premises on which this discussion will rest.

I intend first to discuss treating cases that manifestly involve family problems—such as marital conflicts and parent-child difficulties, to take only two obvious and very common examples—in ways that involve meeting with one or more individual family members separately, during part or all of the treatment, rather than meeting conjointly with the entire family as a fixed principle

---

[1] This is a revised version of a paper presented at the MRI/ETC Conference in Nice, June, 1982. Originally published in the *Journal of Systemic & Strategic Therapies*, (1983), 2 (4).

of therapy—or an unquestioned routine. Secondly, I intend to discuss the treatment of manifestly individual centered presenting problems, such as loneliness and isolation, performance anxieties and difficulties, insomnia, and so on, on the basis of an interactional view of problems, which, as I will explain further shortly, I take as the basic feature of all family therapy. This second topic may be seen as the complement or counterpart of the first.

Two basic premises of the interactional view are fundamental to the treatment approaches to these apparently disparate situations that I will discuss and recommend. Before stating these premises, however, I want to emphasize explicitly that they are just that, premises. That is, I am not claiming to be stating truths or realities about problems and treatment, but simply points of view which I and my colleagues, on the basis of our experience, believe are useful in conceptualizing the nature of problems and their resolution (Weakland, Fisch, Watzlawick, & Bodin, 1974; Watzlawick, Weakland, and Fisch, 1974; Herr and Weakland, 1979; Fisch, Weakland and Segal, 1982). Such premises, essentially, are seen as being parts of a map constructed to guide therapists during the course of therapy; accordingly, they are to be judged on the basis of their usefulness in helping' the therapist and his clients reach the destination of problem resolution.

The first premise is, in my opinion, the most basic feature distinguishing family therapy from most other approaches to psychotherapy (and, indeed, from much of bio-chemical treatment). It rests on taking problems primarily at face value—that is, as consisting of behaviors (usually mentioned in the presenting complaint) which are so disturbed and disturbing yet apparently intractable that someone, seeks professional help in changing them, rather than viewing such behaviors as merely the sign of some deeper and more fundamental disorder in the person or the family. This premise proposes that, at least so far as treatment is concerned, current interaction between the identified patient and involved others is the most central factor in the shaping and maintenance of such problem behavior; and therefore also for its alteration to resolve the problem. While the bases or reasons for this view are not crucial, since, as stated, our adherence to this view rests primarily on the pragmatic criterion of usefulness, some considerations which clarify the relevance and the significance of taking this view seem worth stating. First, the present is all we have to work with. Although the importance of past experience and life history has been stressed in most approaches to psychotherapy, the past is fundamentally a given. It is not subject to change but only, at most, to reinterpretation, which is a present action. Rather similarly, genetic-physiological make-up is also a given whose influence may at most be modifiable by drug dosage—usually an ongoing procedure, and in any case a change imposed by external agency on the passive patient. In marked contrast to this, the interactional viewpoint proposes that present situations, however difficult and distressing they may be, are constantly being remade in the course of present behavior among the individual members of any system. On this view, the persistence of a problem, rather than its origin, is the crucial matter for therapy. Correspondingly, there is always the potential for change in the present—and through this, for the future—by alteration of the behavior of the parties most immediately concerned with the problem, which of course includes their interpretations of both past and current events. Thus, the Interactional View addresses potentials for change rather than limits on it, and sees those involved in problems as responsible actors rather than as passive victims of circumstances—a fundamentally more optimistic and humanistic view of problems.

The second premise is largely a corollary of the first. In simplest terms, it proposes that if interaction between members of a social system is seen as the primary shaper and determinant of ongoing behavior, it then follows that alteration of the behavior of any one member of a system of interaction—particularly a family, as the most ubiquitous, encompassing and enduring kind of system—must lead to a related alteration in the behavior of other members of the system. Accordingly, given sufficient knowledge of interaction in systems, it should be feasible to influence the behavior of any member of a given system indirectly, by influencing the behavior of another member in appropriate respects.

Even if it is recognized that taking the interactional and systemic viewpoint seriously implies that the behavior of any one member can be influenced by altering the behavior of another, however, it would still be reasonable to hold to a standard of meeting conjointly with all members if either of two possible circumstances exist. First, if all of the members are of equal significance for the existence and persistence of the problem, all equally involved, then a standard regime of conjoint meetings might make sense—or at least, there would be no obvious reason to do otherwise. But while there seems to be a common, though largely implicit, assumption among family therapists that this is the case, there are good reasons to be skeptical about any such assumption. A belief in the existence and behavioral importance of interaction among all the members of family (or other) system does not necessarily imply that all interaction within that system is of equal importance for any particular behavior of any member—including any behavior that is labeled as a problem. Indeed, if this were so, therapist addressing any family problem would be overwhelmed from the outset since he would have to consider every behavior observed and reported equally (what a task!) and correspondingly be faced with changing it, all. Instead, and in accord with common observations and knowledge, it makes much more sense to assume that some interactions (and equally, some relationships, since a relationship is mainly a summation or pattern of particular interactions) may be highly significant with respect to certain behaviors by certain persons, but of little relevance for other behaviors or persons. More specifically, some behaviors, or even all the behaviors of some family members, may be of quite peripheral importance for a particular problem behavior of one member. In fact, this is commonly, but implicitly, recognized when a particular school of family therapy assigns primary importance to some selected aspect of family functioning such a "structure" or "communication," and also in the common practice of treating marital problems without the constant involvement of the couples' children in the treatment session.

From this it follows that even when a problem behavior is viewed as basically a response to other behavior in the family context—a view we not only share but promote—this does not imply that the whole family must necessarily be seen it therapy and the whole context of family interaction be investigated and influenced. Rather, there are open questions: What behavior is most significant in the maintenance of the problem, and who needs to be seen and influenced to alter this maintenance and thus resolve the problem?

Even granted this, however, there could still be one reasonable basis for seeing all the family members conjointly. To put it bluntly, if we are ignorant or uncertain about just what family behavior is important in relation to the problem at hand then, although this lack of knowledge is regrettable, it makes certain sense to gather the whole family together. One can observe and question them in hope of gaining some clue as to what aspects of their interaction may be relevant for the existence of the problem; that is, what may need further and more specific inquiry, and if possible, change.

I would suggest that such ignorance and uncertainty were probably significant contributors to the emphasis on seeing the entire family, as a matter of principle, in the early days of family therapy—a principle I myself promoted at one time (Jackson and Weakland, 1961). It was natural and probably inevitable to take this route at a time when our knowledge and position could fairly be summed up as "We are convinced that something in the family context is always important for the existence of a problem, but we are uncertain just what it is, so let us look the family and see if we can find out what is important in the case at hand."

I believe, though, that we have come a long way since those very important, but groping, beginnings. For some years now, my colleagues and I have been structuring treatment in relation to an answer to this question of just what in the family interaction is especially relevant to the existence and persistence of problems. In brief, our view is that problems persist because the efforts of the patient and others concerned to deal with the problem—their attempted solutions—unwittingly serve to maintain or even to exacerbate the problem behavior. Correspondingly, on this view, problem resolution depends on the abandonment of such attempted solutions, and the primary task of the therapist is to promote this particular change of behavior. Since it is difficult to impossible merely to cease any behavior, this usually means that the therapist must promote the substitution of some different and incompatible behavior for the original "solution" behavior. Also, since the original "solution" always appears reasonable and appropriate to those attempting it—it is often a matter of some customary or common sense approach—to produce such change ordinarily will require both active intervention and strategic planning to maximize the therapist's influence. The remainder of this paper will discuss how this view of problems and treatment leads to seeing individual family members separately, and then how it affects dealing with apparently "individual" problems.

Given the general view just stated, the issue of where and how to intervene (like all choices in the course of therapy) becomes a matter of strategic decisions: Who should be seen and influenced in order to interdict the attempted solution most effectively and efficiently; what guidelines are helpful in making this choice, and how can the chosen person or persons best be moved to make such a change?

First and foremost, the therapist should concentrate his efforts on the person who is most concerned about the problem and therefore is most strongly motivated to take action toward change. This person, who may be termed the chief complainant, may or may not be the identified patient. In addition, but secondarily, it may be useful to consider who has most power to instigate change. Just as conceiving the family as a system of relationships involving all the members does not necessarily imply that all members are equally involved in every situation or problem that may occur, it does not imply that they have equal power to maintain or to change things.

These considerations may lead to a focus of attention and effort on some particular individual among those involved in a problem situation, but they are not always important. At times the various participants may be seen, and each influenced to change, at least until the therapist discovers by trial that some particular person is more receptive to his attempts at change than the others. In several common sorts of cases, however, one can recognize at the outset that a certain party to the problem is unlikely to be receptive to intervention toward change while another is likely to be more receptive.

For instance, certain patients come to treatment not on their own initiative and volition, but under duress from others. In all such cases, the therapist's prospects for effecting useful change are much better if he or she can arrange to work primarily with the complainant who instigates treatment rather than with the passive or resistant identified patient. This is most commonly encountered where the identified patient is a child. Very often the child sees no problem existing, except perhaps that his elders are pressuring him unduly. The parents are the complainants and therefore more receptive to making changes if they can be involved in treatment. In addition, they have more power for change in the family than the child—though often they may not realize this initially. Therefore in such cases we work mainly with one or both of the parents. The basic situation is quite similar in other cases of patients under duress, such as one spouse pushed into treatment by the other, or individuals pressed toward treatment by agents of society (teachers, employers, probation officers, judges), although in this last category it may be difficult to establish effective contact with the real complainant.

Another category, which sometimes overlaps the preceding one, involves cases in which one party (often but not always the identified patient) presents him or herself as essentially helpless—willing but unable to carry out any useful actions suggested by a therapist. In such cases, although there are ways of mobilizing the "helpless" person that can be used if necessary, it is often more feasible to work with the "helping" counterpart that ordinarily is present in the situation. For example, a spouse may be distressed by the partner's apparent inadequacy, yet unwittingly supports such behavior by taking over too much responsibility. If the concerned and overly responsible member of the pair can be induced to move away from this position of competent helper; for example, by him or herself engaging in apparently irresponsible statements or actions; this is likely to provide the simplest and most effective resolution of the problem.

A rather different basis for working primarily through an individual—or individuals, separately—exists when parties to a problem are in overt conflict. While this also occurs in many parent-child problems, marital conflict offers the best example of this situation. One conjoint session is often ample to display the typical struggle to the therapist. Further conjoint sessions are likely only to put the therapist into the position of a struggling referee. Even though both parties may sincerely desire change, each wishes the other to do the changing, or at least to change first, and each presses the therapist to take his or her side. In this situation, it is easier and more productive to see one or both of the warring parties alone. When either is seen separately, the therapist can then readily take a commiserating position of agreeing that the individual's spouse is indeed a difficult person to live with—and this may even be true in both cases. Such a position of alliance relaxes that person's defensive posture and sets the stage for acceptance of suggestions for changes in behavior in dealing with the spouse—defined as necessary precisely because such a difficult person requires special handling.

In addition, seeing clients separately may itself demonstrate useful therapeutic points, such as that not all members of a family are of equal status, or that one member's lack of cooperation does not make the others helpless.

Finally, there are cases where a party to a problem just is not directly available; a significant relative living at a distance, or at an identified patient who refuses to see a therapist. Such cases need not end in abandonment or fruitless efforts to bring in the missing party; one can work effectively through whatever concerned person is available.

These general considerations and illustrations of types of case situations provide some guidelines on when to see clients individually rather than conjointly. But when one has decided to see someone individually, what then? That is, within our framework, how does the therapist intervene in order to get the client to substitute some very different behavior, indeed, some opposite behavior if possible, for his attempted solution? This cannot be covered adequately in the present limited compass. Our theory is simple, but its implementation is not:

Effective practice depends on taking account of the particulars, which differs in each case. There is space here only to state some basic principles of such intervention and give an example or two in brief outline.

First, to intervene effectively and rapidly requires that the therapist pay heed to the client's language or position: How does the client view the problem and therapy, and what are the client's beliefs and values? In working briefly, there is no time to teach a client the language and belief system of the therapist, nor do we think this necessary. Our aim is rather to utilize the views and values the client brings to therapy in such a way as to make a significant change, which may appear small, in how the client deals with the problem, in order to interrupt the vicious circle of "problem" and "solution." Four steps are usually involved in doing this:

1. grasping the nature of the client's position;
2. acknowledging and accepting the legitimacy of this view, usually rather explicitly;
3. reframing this view, usually be pointing out special factors in the situation which were not previously taken into account so that the view is given new direction or implication, and
4. utilizing the new direction to propose and promote new and different actions by the client in dealing with the problem.

For example, a parent is concerned about a child's behavior—say, failure to do his school homework adequately—but attributes this failure to an underlying psychological problem, lack of self-confidence. In line with this conception, on the one hand the parent verbally encourages the child ("you can do it") while on the other he or she is always ready to provide help when the child complains of any difficulty with the homework, even if the child does not then utilize such help. It is unlikely that such a parent can effectively be told directly that he or she is supporting the child in being lazy by such leniency and over-helpfulness. More usefully, the therapist could agree with the parent's "diagnosis," but then point out that he or she is inadvertently increasing the child's lack of confidence by making his or her own competence—which is intimidating to the child—too plain both in words ("It's not so hard") and actions (demonstrating competence by helping do the work). Instead, to help the child (a major motivation for the parent) better, he or she should indicate that the work is rather difficult, and while continuing to show willingness to assist, to make errors in helping with the homework which are so obvious that the child will notice them and perhaps even correct the parent. The behavioral aim is to get the parent to stop helping too much and put more responsibility on the child; the means involve the reframing described.

In another case, a wife may complain that her husband doesn't care enough for her, as evidenced by his failure to give her various objects and attentions she personally desires. By cautious inquiry with the wife, and perhaps a session with the husband separately, the therapist determines that she does not tell him what she wants, or at most does so only in vague, unspecific ways, and that the husband would accede to her wishes if he only knew them. In this situation, the therapist avoids trying to point this out to her directly. She is already feeling put down in relation to her husband, and such an attempt would most likely be felt as further blame, and would elicit resistance rather than cooperation. Instead, the therapist can agree that her husband is not treating her as he should, but then reframe this by offering a different reason for his behavior, a reason which puts her one-up on him: It is not that he is uninterested or uncaring about pleasing her. Rather it is that he suffers from a specific deficit; he lacks perceptiveness in emotional matters. Since he is thus sort of mildly retarded in this one sphere, he needs to have whatever she would like made explicit, spelled out to him. On the basis of such reframing, the wife may well be willing to change her behavior in this way, and the problem will be resolved.

As we see it, any limitations to this approach of working with families or couples through one person (or more than one, but separately) are matters of technique rather than of principle. That is, while this approach may not always be the method of choice, there are many situations where it is desirable or necessary, and we see no general contraindications for its use in any sort of problem.

Nevertheless, some cautionary words are necessary. This way of working while simple in principle is complex in practice. As with any therapy, each case is unique in its specific details, which must be taken sufficiently into account. This means especially that adequate and reliable information on the particular case at hand must always be gained as the foundation for any intervention.

While we see this as essential in any form of therapy, it is especially critical when working briefly, and it might seem that there is a risk of inadequate or unreliable information when not all of the parties to a problem may be seen, or not together. This risk is a real, not an imaginary one, but in our experience it is possible to make up for lack of direct observation, by drawing on experience with similar cases where people were seen conjointly, by seeing more than one party separately and comparing their accounts, and most of all by focusing inquiry on what people specifically say and do in relation to the problem, rather than settling for generalities. It is not safe, though, to rely on free use of inference and "perceptiveness" by the therapist in place of careful information gathering.

Now what of "individual problems"? In turning to this topic I am not intending to resurrect the issue, "Can the family view and the individual psychodynamic view be combined, in theory or in practice?" Rather, I intend simply to discuss how my colleagues and I approach various problems that might ordinarily be seen as individual problems—at least manifestly, or by therapists who do not assume every problem is a family problem.

To state the matter briefly, we view and treat all such cases from essentially that same standpoint that I have been outlining before. That is, although in such cases we are more likely to see only one individual (though there are exceptions to this, as will appear), our basic concept is still interactional and our main focus is still on the relationship between the problem behavior and the attempted solution.

There is a sort of transitional class of cases for which the potential applicability of this approach is relatively easy to envision. This class includes those cases where a patient sees a persistent difficulty as his or her own individual problem, but where—to anyone who believes interaction is important in determining behavior—information on the case readily suggests that the behavior of another also is probably relevant to the maintenance of the problem. Such a thought is very likely to arise; for example, in connection with most sexual problems, interaction is rather obviously involved in sexual behavior. The situation is similar in those many problems where a "helper" is involved in trying to cope with the patientts difficulty, as is often the case with problem drinking, for example. The role of interaction may be less evident in anxieties or phobias, but here too a little inquiry will often disclose the existence and importance of someone who helps perpetuate the problem either by encouragement ("You can do it if you try") or by doing for the patient the very things he needs to do for himself, or all too often, both of these.

In fact, the more one looks at this class of cases, the more they seem like any other family therapy cases, except for more emphasis by the patient that it is his or her own, individual problem. (There are counterparts to this also in many problems which family therapists would see as plainly family problems, but are seen differently by the family members, at least initially.) From our viewpoint, this emphasis poses a potential threat to working freely on an interactional basis, but this threatened limitation can be met in either of two ways: In either case the therapist will avoid overt questioning of or arguing with the patient's definition. Then the patient alone may be seen, but interventions are based on the therapist's interactional conception of the problem. Or another relevant person may also be brought into the treatment (seen separately, or possibly conjointly), by defining this other not as a participant in the problem, but simply as someone concerned about it and a possible source of further information or help of some other sort. Otherwise, treatment is much the same as always, that is, focused on interdicting the inappropriate attempted solutions of the patient, of an involved other, or both.

But what about problems that really do seem to involve just the patient, largely or even entirely? For instance, what of the patient who states that his problem is one of extreme social isolation, the patient who has a problem but hides it from everyone but the therapist, apparently successfully, or the patient with insomnia, living alone and simply not discussing it with anyone else?

Even here, we would work according to the same basic model, concerned with how the problem is being handled, the attempted solution. The only significant difference is that in such cases it is the patient's own attempted solutions that are crucial rather than those of anyone else. We still would keep an essentially behavioral view: How does the isolated person act that—again, unwittingly—serves to maintain that isolation? This really takes some doing. Is the hiding of some particular problem, of whatever sort, an important factor in its maintenance? It may well be so; avoidance is a very common attempted solution that perpetuates problems, and conversely, if one can induce a patient to make public announcement of a problem, anxiety or nervousness when speaking, or when meeting a person of the opposite sex, for example, this often is sufficient to resolve the problem.

Also, without straining the concept unduly, one can view even these most "individual" problems interactionally. Just as a person communicates, sometimes loud and clear, by not talking, keeping apart from others is just as interactional as seeking them out. And finally, even the individual grappling alone with a problem, say the insomniac considering and trying out ways to "put himself to sleep," can reasonably be seen as interacting with himself, telling himself what to do, what his solutions should be.

In sum, then, the more one takes the concept of interaction seriously, the less such matters as the particular kind of problem, or the number of persons seen together are definitive of treatment.

# References

Herr, J., and Weakland, J. (1979). *Counseling Elders and Their Families: Practical Techniques for Applied Gerontology.* New York, Springer.

Jackson, D., & Weakland, J. (1961). Family Therapy: Some Considerations on Theory, Technique, and Results, *Psychiatry,* 24 (Supplement to No. 2), 30-45.

Fisch, R., Weakland, J.R., & Segal, L. (1982). *The Tactics of Change: Doing Therapy Briefly.* San Francisco, Jossey-Bass.

Watzlawick, P., Weakland, J., & Fisch, R. (1974). *Change: Principles of Problem Formation & Problem Resolution.* New York, Norton.

Weakland, J., Fisch, R., Watzlawick, P., & Bodin, A. (1974). Brief Therapy: Focused Problem Resolution, *Family Process,* 13, 141-168.

# CHAPTER 13

# The Brief Treatment
# of Alcoholism[1]

*Richard Fisch, M.D.*

## ABSTRACT

*Age-old mystiques and current therapy models about "alcoholics" tend to limit the scope of research on abusive drinking. A non-pathologic, non-normative model formulated by the Brief Therapy Center of MRI is offered as a possibility for expanding directions of research. The model and its application to abusive drinking is illustrated by a case description.*

Excessive uses of behavior altering substances have always been surrounded by a mystique and this certainly has been the case for alcohol. Prior to the late nineteenth century and the invention of "mental illness" drunkenness had been considered a work of the devil or a peculiar defect of character setting the drunkard apart from the mainstream of his or her society. The "town drunk" was a unique character, an object of ridicule or amusement and often the prime example of waywardness in the minister's sermons to his congregation. Concomitantly, magical qualities were attributed to alcohol itself, a fiendish invention of the devil to tempt the weak into his control; "the evils of drink." The fact that the vast bulk of the drinking population had no problem

[1] Originally published in the *Journal of Systemic & Strategic Therapies, (1986).* 5: 3; 40-49

in using alcohol made little difference *in* these mystical attributions about drunkards and alcohol and, for that matter, these concepts played a significant part in the Constitutional amendment known as "Prohibition."

Beginning in the mid-nineteenth century, many forms of deviance were explained as being caused by an illness, and, in particular, an illness of the mind. Originally intended as a metaphor allowing for the humane treatment of the "mad" and to offset the brutalizing typified by "Bedlam," the metaphor came to be regarded as fact and ushered in the era of what is currently called "mental illness" and the "mental health movement."

Because of the moral judgments made about excessive drinking, it was slower to catch up with other forms of deviance in being viewed as a "mental illness" rather than characterilogical weakness or sin. I think more than any professional developments, the creation of Alcoholics Anonymous did the roost in legitimizing excessive drinking as a "disease" and thereby endowing "alcoholics" with the uneasy respectability accorded other forms of deviance that had graduated from "badness" to "illness." For good or bad, however, the in-grouping of drinkers inherent in the social organization of A. A. has tended to confirm the traditional concept that the excessive user of alcohol *is* a "breed apart" from the mainstream of the general population, and in recent years, this has extended to the families of A.A. members with the creation of Alanon and Alateen organizations.

Despite the humanizing of "treatment" of the drinker, traditional psychiatric models, as well as the model of A. A., continued to view alcoholism as stemming from a basic defect within the individual, a defect so intrinsic to the problem drinker that "curing" the drinker is not regarded as possible; "once an alcoholic always an alcoholic," regardless of extended periods of sobriety. Much as schizophrenia is regarded, the sober drinker is an "alcoholic in remission." This, of course, is clearly and firmly supported by the model used in A.A. in which excessive drinking is regarded as the manifestation of an inherent "allergy to alcohol" and it is explicitly emphasized to members that to risk one drink is to be thrown back into the depths of uncontrolled drinking.

In the nineteen fifties, a different conceptualization evolved to explain deviance, the application of cybernetic principles, "systems." Thus, the individual was no longer viewed as having or being the problem, but rather the "symptom bearer" of the integrated unit, usually the family unit. Further, it was explained that the "system," be it molecular, animal or human, required stereotyped interactions to maintain a stability of the system for its ongoing functioning, or "homeostasis;" and in some units or families, a stereotypical interaction might be the performance of and encouragement of (usually covert) what would be regarded as symptomatic behavior—*i.e.* the "dysfunctional homeostasis" of that family. Not the individual, but the family as an organization "needed" the "symptom." Finally, in order to eliminate (cure, modify, resolve) the symptom, it would require some fundamental reorganization of the family's "homeostasis." It was, and still is in many quarters, believed that simply attempting to remove the symptom would either not work (since the "system" would resist attempts to change it), or possibly worse, a new problem and/or a new "identified patient" would arise to reconstitute the former "dysfunctional homeostasis." In brief, the newer "systems" concepts introduced a departure from traditional "monadic" views but retained the concept of "pathology," a new variant on the "iceberg theory" that the problem is the tangible expression of an underlying (hidden, covert, unconscious, unaware, deep seated) process or structure supporting and maintaining that symptom.

The staff at the Brief Therapy Center have, for about the past 18 years, been applying a different model, having as a major feature that it is not pathology oriented  principally, that regardless of how problems arise, they are maintained by the very efforts the "afflicted" and/or others involved in the problem are making to attempt to resolve it. It is not an article of faith that the individual or family needs the problem, nor that there is anything wrong with them that they persist in problem maintaining "solutions" but the belief that one is inclined to be trapped by one's frame of reference and will continue to do what is "logical" regardless of the failure of those efforts. ("If at first you don't succeed, try, try again" and again, and again.) Secondly, the model is non-normative and importance is not attached to standards of "mental health," "functional family homeostasis" and the like. Instead, it is a complaint-based model, the standard for entering into "treatment" that someone is registering a complaint (about oneself or another) and the standard for terminating "treatment" that the complainant no longer has that complaint. (For further description of the model see Fisch, Weakland, & Segal, 1982; Watzlawick, Weakland, & Fisch, 1974; Weakland, Fisch, Watzlawick, & Bodin, 1974.)

This model has a bearing on the way staff at the Brief Therapy Center go about the treatment of any problem including that of "alcoholism." Since it is a non-pathologic model, we cannot, logically, view the excessive drinker as having a unique vulnerability to alcohol nor, for that matter, that the family has any investment, needed or otherwise, in maintaining an excessive drinker. Thus we can, in fact must, consider that the resolution of that problem can be relatively brief since it, like all other problems, is actively maintained by the unwitting, albeit problem maintaining, efforts of the parties involved; that interdicting those efforts can and should result in the self extinction of the problem. Additionally, as a non-pathologic model, there is no reason to regard as unfeasible that an excessive drinker can become a "normal" drinker, or "social drinker" and that it is likely that the rarity of this outcome is of twofold reasons: first, that extant models require, logically, abstinence as the only possible resolution and therefore too little effort has been made in attempting otherwise, and secondly, that in those few attempts to bring about controlled drinking, the models and/or techniques used have been inappropriately applied.

The following is an account of a case of "alcoholism" treated at the Brief Therapy Center which can better illustrate how we would go about this kind of problem. It is not being offered as proof of the feasibility of brief treatment for drinking nor of the feasibility of converting an "alcoholic" into a social drinker. It is offered to exemplify our approach and that successful brief treatment of excessive drinking is possible.

Lucy, a 33 year old married woman and part-time piano teacher and mother of two young children, called our Center saying she needed help for her drinking problem. On the phone she said that her husband Jack, an accountant, was also concerned about her drinking but that she was seeking help on her own, and not from any coercion on his part. Because both were concerned about the problem, we would have wanted to meet with them both but his schedule, at the time, precluded his coming in and rather than delay treatment, we decided to go ahead and meet with her alone for that first session.

In that session, she said that she has been drinking *to* excess for about 5 years, usually wine, and mostly in the evenings and nights, often consuming a fifth during the evening hours. On many nights she was in a semi-drunken state collapsing into bed, or on the couch, long after her husband had retired. She added that her drinking had significantly eroded her social life and the productive use of daytime hours and had been a factor in the alienation from her husband, especially sexually. When it began to affect her health she became alarmed enough to seek treatment about two years ago. Her physician told her she was showing definite signs of liver damage and this, in turn, had affected her hormonal system so that her periods became very irregular. She added that in the last 4 months her periods had stopped altogether.

Because she was a woman of great pride, she resented and rejected the idea that she was "too weak" to be able to control her drinking and chose a therapist who offered her the possibility of becoming a controlled drinker. For the most part, her therapist attempted to achieve this by emphasizing her responsibility for her drinking, by encouraging her to take conscious and deliberate control over her intake and/or periods of abstinence, to use substitutes for alcohol such as herb teas and use as a basic guideline "choosing or not choosing to drink." However, after two years of treatment her drinking, if anything, was worse and after a humiliating confrontation with her parents she felt she had to admit the treatment was not working. Her therapist concurred with her request to seek treatment elsewhere and gave her a number of names for referral, including ours. Because she had spent two years in therapy, she was attracted by the idea that our Center dealt with problems on a brief basis. Although she said that controlled drinking seemed to be unfeasible for her she nevertheless, emphasized that resolving her problem through abstinence was a surrendering to an image of weakness akin to being a disabled person. Since we see controlled drinking as a viable possibility, we held open that option to her but in a way that would not commit her solely to that option. We told her that while it was possible for some "alcoholics" to become social drinkers, this was rare and that she should understand that if she were still hoping for that kind of resolution it would be significantly more difficult and that it required a person of exceptional strength of character to achieve it further, that it was unlikely she was that exceptional and that it might be better for her to direct her efforts toward abstinence as most "alcoholics" do.

She said she understood that and her re-gearing to see a new therapist was with the expectation that she needed to learn to stay away from alcohol. However, she said that the idea of controlling her drinking was still very strong with her, and despite the failure in that attempt over the last two years, she was still hoping that she could be "strong enough" to "master" her drinking rather than admit it had mastered her.

We met with her husband in the second session, and as is our custom when we have seen a spouse even once alone, we saw him alone for that session. He confirmed much of what Lucy had said about the course of the problem, her prior treatment and the impact of her drinking on him and their marriage. He added some further information, mainly the directives the previous therapist had given him: to "make Lucy's drinking her problem, not his" and that he should implement that idea by walking out of the room when she is drinking or drunk and avoid giving her lectures about drinking. He said he had done his best to cooperate but in seeing no change, or her drinking worsening, it was difficult to be detached about it and he continued to make critical comments to her, usually in a snide or offhanded manner or take her to task the next day after a drunken bout. He also discouraged her from social contacts in which there would likely be drinking and this cut down their social life since they rarely went to parties but also avoided less formal social engagements with friends who were big on drinking. He also found it difficult to avoid monitoring her drinking in other ways—checking for hidden bottles or the level of wine in bottles, assessing her state of sobriety or insobriety when he came home from work. In that latter regard, if he felt her speech was at all slurred or her eyes slightly glassy or she was unduly irritable, he concluded she was drunk or well on the way and he would plan on spending the evening avoiding her in an effort to detach himself and give some semblance of cooperation with the therapist's directives.

After that session, the treatment team assessed the data we had gotten from Lucy and her husband, Jack. First, it was clear that *both* were complainants, and despite the unease in their marriage, were in accord that it was very important to resolve the drinking problem. Secondly, in all the efforts they had made and in the suggestions her therapist had given them, they appeared to be variations on a central theme, different as they might appear on the surface. That central theme was that in order to resolve her drinking problem, it was necessary that she be on constant guard, i.e. preoccupied. For example, since she was present at the session her therapist had suggested the husband leave the room when he was angry with her drinking, his leaving the room would have to take on a new significance and instead of it being an act of "detachment" it would be a silent, but pointed comment on her drinking, and ironically, his continued absence from the room (usually the living room) would be a constant reminder of her drinking. Similarly, if she drank some herbal tea, the tea would remind her what it was a substitute for. At those times when she would set herself a period of abstinence, say a month or so, she would have to think about "not drinking," but thereby, think about drinking. In its essence, the "attempted solution" became an ever increasing spiral of preoccupation in which efforts to avoid drinking, promoted by her or her husband or her therapist, escalated this preoccupation about alcohol.

Our overall strategy then, was to interdict Lucy's preoccupation with drinking and we believed this might be accomplished if we could prevent her husband from continuing to be an outspoken or silent reminder of her drinking. Since he was accustomed to checking on her presumed state of insobriety each evening and on weekends, we thought this afforded the best focal point to intervene in and we thought we could most effectively intervene by creating doubt in his mind about the reliability of his assessment.

Thus, in session three, we met with both and explaining that whatever way they might resolve the problem, it would be important for him to be "perceptive" of her level of drinking, partly as a way of checking progress and as a safeguard when things might slip back. However, we continued, we weren't sure how perceptive he was since accuracy was very important. Therefore, as a next step in treatment, his perceptivity needed to be checked out. To do this, Lucy was instructed to randomize her quantity of drinking from day to day and to keep a secret record of exactly how much she had drunk on any day. At the same time, she was to randomize her demeanor sober or intoxicated-wise—especially when he came home in the evening. He then was to make his best assessment of how much she had drunk and to keep his own secret record of that each day. They were then to bring in their records so we could compare them, and thereby, assess how accurate or inaccurate his perceptivity was. If the intervention was to work, there would have to be a significant disparity in their separate records. In such a case, this would likely engender doubt in his continuing efforts to draw any conclusions about her drinking levels, hopefully to the point that he would regard it as an exercise in futility and not bother to monitor her, but instead, go on about his business, thus becoming more casual about her drinking.

However, his estimate of her drinking levels was so close to the mark on most every day there was no credible way of indicating a significant disparity. Ironically, on the one day his estimate was way off, Lucy piped up in the session to say that that was the day she wasn't sure how much she had had and that Jack was probably correct in his estimate. While nothing was gained from this intervention, it did not lose anything since the purported reason for the task was simply to check on his perceptivity. Thus, we concluded that session by saying that we were reassured about him.

Since that effort got "shot down," the team had to plan on a different tactical approach, however, one still involving Jack. We thought we could achieve the same blocking of his "watchdog" position if we could have him shift to a position of openly encouraging her drinking, and at the same time, put *her* in the position of controlling her drinking, not under pressure from him, but in *resistance* to his encouraging her to drink we hoped that the success of this intervention would be enhanced by the attractiveness to Lucy of being "one-up" on Jack by controlling her drinking rather than feeling she had "knuckled under" and being more "one-down" to him. We also realized we had a prior task with them, especially Jack, since the intervention would be one of controlled drinking, something he considered impossible and a lost cause.

In session 5 we reconfirmed with Lucy that she still very much hoped to resolve her drinking problem through controlled drinking rather than abstinence. We reiterated our position that this was very unlikely, but because of her resolve, that issue had to be dealt with so that she could get that hope out of her way and address herself more committedly to the tasks of abstinence. As we hoped, her husband accepted that rationale and we were able to turn our attention to the intervention we had in mind, which was framed as a way of giving Lucy the opportunity to prove, once and for all, that she could resolve her problem through control, or if not, she would have to forget it. We emphasized that control of one's drinking was not the same as trying to drink as little as possible but rather that one could, on any day, target a desired level of drinking and be able to "hit" that target, no more no less. We added that in order to achieve that difficult ability, it would be necessary for Lucy to do it "the hard way," i.e. not only for Jack not to support her in her endeavor but to provide obstacles and resistance to it. Also, in that way, should she be able to achieve her unlikely goal, it would be clear to both of them that she had truly mastered her drinking by doing it without support. Again, both were agreeable to that rationale.

In practice, she was to set a targeted goal of drinking each day, a level she felt she could handle. He however, was to try to tempt her to exceed it in any way he could devise, obviously or subtly. For example, we suggested that he call her at unexpected times during the day and ask that she take a drink or to suggest it on weekends when he was home. We asked them to return in two weeks to give this "program" a fuller trial.

When they came in they said that they had embarked on the task and had kept it up most of that first week, but after that, had abandoned it. Their reason for doing that was ironic: he had forgotten to call one day, and Lucy angrily, defined that as his reneging on the agreement. In her anger she said that since he had reneged, she didn't want to pursue it any longer either. He took her at her word but she failed to inform him that after she had cooled down, she had changed her mind and decided to get back to it. Jack then didn't bother to call anymore, and Lucy took this as confirmation that he wasn't interested in pursuing the program. As a temporizing step, we defined their actions as an "unconscious" but mutually coordinated effort to sabotage a program that possibly could have led to the resolution of her drinking problem, and a resolution of the most desired way, through controlled drinking. With that framing we shifted to the agenda of "the dangers of improvement." "Had we," they and us, "been obtuse to the *disadvantages* of resolving their problem?" we explained; and had their collective unconscious "wisely" alerted us to this possibility? (As a note to the reader, the foregoing formulation is nothing more than an *explanation* given to the couple to convey that when they agree to carry out a task or suggestion, but then fail to follow through on it, we take that seriously, and at least temporarily, put further efforts to resolve their problem "on hold." It is one alternative to something we believe is counterproductive which is to urge, exhort or cajole people to carry out a previously agreed on task. Consistent with the non-pathologic element of our model, we do not view failures to "do their homework" as an expression of "sabotage" or "needing the symptom" but rather as carelessness or half-heartedness, or at times, misunderstanding the assignment.)

The remainder of that session was spent in exploring some possible disadvantages of resolving the problem and they themselves came up with a few. For example, Jack said that while he was very discomfited by her drinking, it was consistent enough so that some of her behavior was predictable. If, on the other hand, she either stopped drinking or became a controlled drinker, he might be in an apprehensive state wondering, each day, if that improvement might break down. We offered another one we felt would especially appeal to Lucy: in her current "alcoholic" state, it would be easier for Jack to discount her opinions on many issues, while as a sober person and one who had over come a difficult condition, he would have to acknowledge the legitimacy of her ideas even when they disagreed with his, and that he might find it a problem to adjust to a relationship in which he could not easily be "one-up." They were sent home with the task of thinking more about the possible disadvantages of improvement since "no further steps should be taken to resolve the problem until we can assess those dangers and evaluate whether they might be better off just leaving things as they are." As is customary with such an assignment and because of the reasons for that type of intervention, we asked that they meet with us in two weeks rather than one. (This echoes the implicit message that we are putting problem solving on hold while affording them an opportunity to recoup from their previous delinquency by doing a different "homework.")

In the next session, number 7, they came back with notes on the thinking and discussion they had done, and had been able to come up with an additional number of "dangers of change," i.e. they had done their homework well. The therapist felt that the point had been well made, and as planned, decided to shift to an assignment intended to interdict their attempted solution. At that point, he acknowledged that there were considerable dangers in resolving the problem, and he therefore, wanted to take time out to consult with his colleagues. In that ad hoc conference, two things were decided: that the therapist would appear to be the lone dissenting voice in the team in opposition to his colleagues' unanimous opinion that resolving the problem would create more and worse problems than it solved. Secondly, we all believed that their fumbling with the previous suggestion meant that it would not be an appropriate tactic, and even if carried out by them, would likely result in too partial a resolution. (We were to learn later that we had underestimated them, especially Jack.) Therefore, the "dissenting" therapist was to suggest a different task, albeit one based on the same overall strategy of the treatment, i.e. to get Jack to back off from being her "watchdog" about drinking, as well as interdict Lucy's own ways of remaining preoccupied about drinking.

On returning to the treatment room, the therapist reported that he was the lone voice believing that while there were significant dangers to resolving their problem, they could handle those dangers and overcome them, and thus, he was prepared to go ahead with treatment and face his colleagues' opprobrium and pessimism. He then outlined the program for them: Lucy was to set for herself a level of drinking each day that she believed she could handle. If on any day she exceeded that level, she was to inform Jack. He then was instructed to go to the store on Saturday morning, buy two bottles of the wine Lucy usually drank, pour all of one bottle into an appropriate number of glasses, and sitting at the dining table, he was to insist she drink them, one by one, until that whole fifth was consumed. Then, they were to do the same thing with the second bottle on Sunday morning. She was instructed not to "guzzle" that quantity of alcohol, but to take her time even if it took all day. In any case, they were not to do anything else until that task was completed each day. If, however, she did not exceed her limit on any day during the week, she was not required to go through this "treatment," and in fact, would be allowed to drink as much or as little on the weekend as she pleased; it was "off time." They agreed to do it and we felt that a two week trial would be more appropriate than one week.

Before they returned for session number 8, the treatment team had tried to anticipate as many possibilities of the outcome of the assignment as we could entertain: they changed their minds and decided not to do it; they tried doing it but flubbed that too; they "misinterpreted" the assignment; they did it and well but discounted any change resulting from it; and so on. But, as Burns has said "... the best laid plans of mice and men often go awry," and we, as well as the clients had not foreseen what obstructed the assignment: in the interim, Lucy had gone for a follow-up check to her gynecologist who announced to her that she was pregnant; four months pregnant as a matter of fact! When Lucy told him of the assignment, he said that the level of the enforced drinking, should she need to do it, could harm the fetus and he suggested that she hold off until we could discuss it with her, and if need be, him.

We definitely agreed with that caution and planned to talk directly with the gynecologist to confirm the opinion Lucy had conveyed for him. Under the circumstances, the session was a short one, but we did discuss some alternative possibilities, assuming that any planned excessive drinking would have to be eliminated. Any alternatives were very general and the session was left on the uncertain note of: "We'll talk to your doctor and, assuming your understanding is correct, I and my colleagues will confer and see what might be the next best step." A light note was lent to the session, realizing that in her earlier report that her periods had stopped, none of us had thought of a natural and obvious reason.

Her gynecologist did confirm what Lucy had reported. Interestingly, he said that since she is inclined to be a "nervous" person, moderate drinking would be of some benefit during the pregnancy, but he did not view her as capable of doing that, since he was aware of her "alcoholic" problem. Mainly, he cautioned against any deliberate excessive consumption and we readily agreed with that opinion. In our conference, the team was in a quandary: apparently, none of the previous interventions had worked (we were to learn differently in the next session), or they were fumbled. To make matters more difficult, there were only two sessions left in our ten session limit. Considering the constraints we had and the clients were under, we believed that the use of those two sessions could best be spent in seeing Jack alone and focusing on his "watchdog" position. We also believed that at that point in treatment, we could be more direct with him in relating his efforts to stop Lucy from drinking with the very difficulty she was having in overcoming her preoccupation with drinking and succumbing to that preoccupation.

Therefore, we saw Jack alone in session 9, and it was to be the last session. Before taking up the agenda we had in mind, we realized that we had been so busy devising interventions, that we had not taken time to check with them on the state of the problem, and so we began the session by asking him what had been happening with her drinking. This was when we realized we had underestimated him.

He said that in the month preceding the Christmas holiday, she had done very well. She was quite temperate in her drinking, never overdid it, and he was amazed at her control. During the holidays, however, she slipped and became intoxicated a few times. He reported that this made him apprehensive and that he found himself going back to his customary "watchdog" position, checking on her state of sobriety, counting drinks, etc. He added that from the earliest of sessions, he had understood that his "watchdogging" played an integral part in her drinking and regardless of the fumbling about interventions, he had on his own, resolved to back off from that former position, but admitted that with her excessive drinking during the holidays, that resolve dissipated. However, he had decided to back off again, and her drinking, accordingly, diminished significantly. He finished by saying that in observing the interaction between his "watchdogging" and her drinking, he was convinced of the interplay between the two, and he hoped he would not slip again. The therapist told him it might not be necessary for him to be ever watchful about himself. It might suffice if he simply told Lucy that he had come to realize the counterproductivity of his keeping a surveillance on her, but that since it was an old habit, he might slip, from time to time, despite his best intentions, and that when he did, he would appreciate her letting him know so he could be more aware of it and drop it. It was mutually agreed that, while there was one session left, it would be better to leave that last appointment ad hoc should the need arise.

As is our custom in all treatments, an evaluation was done three months and one year after the last appointment. In the 3 month evaluation, Lucy said she felt she had her drinking under control, attributing some of that to the pleasant anticipation of the baby's arrival and concern for its welfare. No other problems had arisen nor were any other problems not dealt with at the Center improved and there had been no further treatment. Jack's comments echoed hers: that she had markedly controlled her drinking and that he found it easier to stay away from being a "watchdog."

At the one-year follow-up Lucy said she felt she was still controlling her drinking and that there had been no further treatment. The baby, she added, was healthy and had suffered no ill effects from her drinking in the earliest trimester of the pregnancy. Jack's assessment was less enthusiastic. He said that he felt her control of drinking was not as good as it had been, "about 60% of what it was" during the latter part of treatment and the several months after, but that it was so much better than before treatment, he wasn't sure if he should be apprehensive. He said he had been thinking of coming in to see us but did not feel it imperative at that point. He was told that if he should feel it necessary or even useful that we would be glad to see him and could do that without much delay. He did not call us back and so we assumed that his anxieties had abated.

This article and the case illustration is not intended as a compelling argument for the brief treatment of "alcoholism" nor that resolution of that problem can convert excessive drinkers into controlled drinkers. It is instead, intended as encouragement to researchers and clinicians to pursue continued efforts to investigate those possibilities. In our limited experience it can be done, however uncommon so far, and it is all the more significant since the professional and lay climate is strongly discouraging to "alcoholics" to entertain such possibilities; discouragement on the explicit, and more importantly, on the implicit level, as Lucy's previous therapist had conveyed (e.g. suggesting that Lucy would need substitutes to replace her "need" *for* drinking, while on the explicit level, supporting her wish to attempt controlled drinking).

Finally, the article is intended to illustrate and explicate the model used at the Brief Therapy Center, and its strategic and tactical application to a problem of substance abuse, so that the reader can be clear about that model and its application, and can make clearer comparisons with other systemic and strategic models.

## References

Fisch, R., Weakland, J., and Segal, L. (1982). *The Tactics of Change - Doing Therapy Briefly*, Jossey-Bass, San Francisco.

Watzlawick, P., Weakland, J., and Fisch, R. (1974). *Change: Principles of Problem Formation and Problem Resolution*, W.W. Norton, New York.

Weakland, J., Fisch, R., Watzlawick, P., and Bodin, A. (1974). "Brief Psychotherapy – Focused Problem Resolution," *Family Process,* 13: 147-168.

# CHAPTER 14

# Cases That "Don't Make Sense":
## Brief Strategic Treatment in Medical Practice[1]

### John H. Weakland and Richard Fisch

*Brief, strategic, family-oriented approaches are particularly suited to a number of the problems seen in primary care medicine. Careful history-taking often makes evident ways in which apparently un-understandable behavior in fact makes sense. Of particular interest are the ways in which efforts to change unwanted behavior operate to sustain and maintain it. A logical intervention plan can then be devised that provides family members with acceptable alternate behaviors that do not maintain the symptom.*

As they should be, physicians in family practice are usually the first professional recourse for most families encountering any somatic—and many psychosomatic—difficulties. In the course of this, however, primary care physicians are often presented with problems that "don't make sense" as standard medical problems, and in ways that make diagnosis and treatment puzzling and difficult.

A relatively simple example of such a situation—though not necessarily simple to deal with—might involve a man who is found by his physician to have hypertension. Conventional treatment, including hypertensive medication, dietary changes, and avoidance of stress are prescribed. However, after

---

[1] This article is adapted from a chapter originally published in S. Henao & N. Grose, (Eds.) , (1985). *Principles of family systems in family medicine.* New York: Brunner/Mazel.

brief initial improvement, blood pressure levels continue to be elevated, although the patient reports that he is faithfully adhering to the medical regimen, and no physiological defects can be found to account for the problem.

In a more extreme example, an obese mother brings an obviously overweight child to the doctor with the complaint that "he doesn't eat," and insists that this is the problem, angrily brushing aside the doctor's attempts to suggest that, if anything, the child must be overeating. Or another mother brings her child because he is passing black stools. On careful examination, the physician finds that the child is basically quite healthy, but this does not allay the mother's concern, and the symptom persists (Henao, 1982).

Other examples, while less blatantly confusing, still involve situations difficult to understand and deal with effectively: A man comes for his physical checkup accompanied by his wife. She exhibits marked concern about his physical condition, but the patient himself appears strangely passive, unconcerned, and uncooperative-he gives minimal information, discounts the seriousness of any findings, and so on. Or a young man comes in complaining of vague symptoms and, despite negative physical findings and reassurance by the physician, remains uneasy and insists on further tests.

Without claiming to be exhaustive, several kinds of such puzzling and difficult situations that one is apt to meet fairly often in family practice can be listed:

1. The problem appears to be an ordinary one, but the patient's (or a concerned relative's) complaint persists after standard treatment is applied—either the signs and symptoms continue, or the complaint persists despite objective evidence of amelioration or resolution of the physical problem.
2. The complaint does not make sense to the physician from the outset. This can occur in several ways:
   a. Information given is so vague or inadequate that diagnosis is very difficult.
   b. Information given by the patient and/or family members is contradictory, so that there is no clear picture of the problem.
   c. The patient's, or family's, statements are clear enough, but they do not fit with the physician's observations and medical knowledge; this may concern either the nature or the severity of the complaint.

Such puzzling situations, we suggest, often result from the fact that in addition to physical factors, family factors may play a considerable part in the nature, genesis, and resolution of complaints brought to family physicians. In emphasizing the frequent existence and importance of such family factors in the practice of family medicine, we are not aiming to further complicate the tasks facing the family physician. Rather, we are proposing that such factors simply exist. Like it or not, they are inherently involved in medical practice, and understanding them can aid in handling them effectively and therefore "uncomplicate" treatment.

## The Family as Case Environment

Viewing the medical patient in the context of his or her family is a useful conceptual tool available to all physicians. While it is not a necessary concept for the continuation of the physician's duty to the patient, its utility lies in affording the interested physician a means whereby he can expand the range of effectiveness with his patients and, at the same time, make his work more efficient. Nor is the view of the patient-in-the-context-of-the-family totally new in medicine. It is, after all, an extension of the tradition of viewing the patient in this environment, in which the family is seen as a significant part.

Let us use an analogy: A physician can correctly diagnose a case of lead poisoning and apply appropriate treatment for the ultimate reduction of lead levels in the blood. However, he will not be satisfied with the treatment until the *source* of the poisoning—perhaps lead in a water pipe—is identified, since continuing contamination of the patient will only make his best treatment efforts a futile attempt to stem the tide. In similar fashion, the family of the medical patient, in their interactions, can influence each other's health and compliance with treatment for good or bad. Thus, in our first example, the patient's wife may be acting in some way that unwittingly provokes stress and anxiety in him, contributing—like the lead in the water pipe—to a continuation of the problem, so that it can only be resolved by dealing with this source of trouble.

Family factors were also involved, though in rather more complex ways, in our other examples. Maternal anxiety and accompanying distortion of perception or evaluation were basic to the next two cases mentioned above. In the first of these, the mother was so anxious that her son eat "enough," and so over-controlling in her attempts to ensure this, that she provoked some discernible resistance by her son. Although he still overate, this resistance then became to her an unquestionable sign that he was "not eating," a sign more significant for her than his weight or appearance. In the other example, it was discovered that the mother was concerned that her child was "sickly," so she had been giving him iron pills to "build his strength"—thus the black stools. In the next case the husband and wife were involved in a covert, and possibly unrecognized, struggle for control, which was being played out in terms of nurturance and concern for his health on her part, met by him with passive resistance and rejection of any proposed basis for such concern. And in the final example, it turned out that the young man's anxieties, expressed as somatic concerns, were largely based on having doubts, which he was reluctant to face directly, about his approaching marriage.

## When Family Factors Matter

While the family is relevant for all cases a family physician sees, there are of course many instances where this presents no treatment problem. When the patient and family members are reasonably informative and cooperative, and there is a clear physical problem, family factors need no special attention. Several common sorts of situations can be identified, however, in which deliberate attention to family interaction is likely to be important or even crucial. In the first place, it is well-known that many of the common miseries for which the family physician is usually the first recourse—anxiety, tension, depression, insomnia, for example—are as likely to be psychological or behavior problems as strictly physiological ones. In all such cases the family is highly pertinent because it forms a major part of the environment within which the individual patient is functioning poorly.

Next, there are the many problems now classified as "psychosomatic," where a relationship is recognized between an evident physiological dysfunction and the psychological functioning of the individual patient. Since the individual's psychological state is highly dependent on family interaction—an obvious potential source of stress as well as support—the family situation needs to be taken into account more than has been customary in such cases. Indeed, we have proposed that this territory might better be called "family somatics" (Weakland, 1977). It is also conceivable that certain kinds of interaction may lead to, or at least potentate, susceptibility to infectious agents or physiological abnormality, since we do not yet know how far interactional influence may extend into physiological functioning. That is, family interaction may have relevance even for clearly medical diseases, not just interpersonal or psychological ones. This, however, is more a matter for research in the long term than of medical practice in the here and now.

Also, it may happen that an apparently physical problem is primarily an unanticipated and unfortunate, but direct, consequence of family behavior. Henao's example (1982), mentioned earlier, of the young child passing black stools is a case in point. Or, more commonly, family concern about an aging member's infirmities may lead to that person taking too much medication, or too many kinds, until confusion develops, which may then be viewed simply as senile dementia. This example also suggests that by withholding relevant information, applying direct or subtle pressure for inappropriate treatment, and so on, the family as well as the physician may play a significant role even in some apparently "iatrogenic" disorders.

Thus, family interaction may be important in the origin of a problem brought to the physician. It will certainly be significant for the medical handling of any case. When family interaction is for the better, there is no problem, but the physician needs to be alert to the fact that it may often be for the worse: family factors can profoundly influence initiation or delay of treatment, how seriously a symptom is regarded, how well the patient cooperates with the physician and treatment program, and how satisfied the patient is with the outcome of treatment.

All of this is really not new. Practicing family physicians have long been aware that anxiety and tension can be rooted in a family or marital relationship, that some patients or family members minimize problems while others exaggerate them, and that patients and their family members (who are inescapably involved in any illness and treatment) may be non-cooperative, cooperative, or even over-cooperative. Physicians once absorbed knowledge about the medical significance of the family, and about how to deal with this aspect of practice, by prolonged direct contact with whole families. Today, this is seldom feasible. Meanwhile, family therapists and associated family systems researchers have been accumulating knowledge about family interaction and its powerful influence in determining the behavior and functioning of individual members that can usefully be extended and applied in the practice of family medicine.

In short, we are only proposing to outline and exemplify how family physicians can take family factors which are inherent in their practice into account more systematically and effectively—much as physical factors are explored and dealt with systematically rather than piecemeal and ad hoc in modern medicine.

It is plain that family therapists vary considerably in their particular emphases and approaches. We believe the strategic approach developed at the Brief Therapy Center of the Mental Research Institute (Fisch, Weakland, & Segal 1982; Herr & Weakland, 1979; Watzlawick, Weakland, & Fisch, 1974) is especially relevant for wider application to family practice. Some approaches to the family are so broad or comprehensive that, while they may be useful in obtaining an overall view of family functioning, they are very time-consuming for a busy practitioner and much of the information gathered may be of little relevance to the particular medical complaint at hand. In contrast, our approach is more narrowly focused on how the family is involved in the current problem and its treatment, in the here and now. While an adequate medical history of the problem is of course necessary, in our approach there is no need for gathering all family members to seek an overall view of family structure and functioning or family history, nor do we see either general family reorganization or basic personality change of individuals as needed for successful treatment.

Only certain limited information needs to be gathered, and limited behavioral changes encouraged.

## Focal Aspects of the Strategic Approach

Our approach focuses explicitly on: 1. clarifying the presenting complaint; 2. investigating what factors in the patient and family promote the persistence of the complaint, especially attempted "solutions" by the patient and others that only keep things had, or even worsen them; 3. identification of what changes seem needed to resolve the complaint; and 4. determining effective means to promote these changes. We may now consider how these foci are important not just in family psychotherapy, but apply equally and similarly in family medical practice, where puzzling cases are likely to present difficulties in the following: a. diagnosis—forming a clear picture of the presenting problem; b. formulating what needs to be done to resolve or ameliorate this problem, either by direct treatment or by appropriate referral; c. obtaining patient and family cooperation to ensure that this *is* done; or some combination of these.

1. The presenting complaint of course is not everything, either in strategic family therapy or in family practice, and is not necessarily to be taken at face value. It may largely be a sign of some underlying problem that needs alteration or correction. It may, as several of the initial examples illustrate, be a cover or substitute for a problem of a different sort. In addition, there may not be a correlation between the "seriousness" of someone's complaint and the related physiological, psychosomatic, or behavioral problem when judged from a detached, objective standpoint. A patient or family member may not show appropriate concern about a serious health problem, or conversely may show excessive concern about something minor. Any of these situations pose complexities and obstacles to effective diagnosis and treatment, and can understandably be irritating to a concerned and busy practitioner.

Despite all this, the presenting complaint is highly important in several respects. It is the starting point, the matter that brings the patient to treatment, and the center of the patient's (or the family's) interest and concern. It therefore must be accepted and taken seriously, at least overtly, in order to initiate that cooperative relationship between physician and patient on which any effective treatment depends. Similarly, the status of the presenting complaint is crucial for termination of treatment and evaluation of its outcome. No matter what has been objectively accomplished in regard to the patient's health and functioning, the patient or family will usually not be *satisfied* unless the complaint has somehow been resolved. Otherwise, there will likely be continued demands for treatment, even though the physician deems this unnecessary from a strictly physical standpoint.

It is therefore especially important in all difficult or confusing cases—even those in which a medical diagnosis is clear from physical examination and history—to get a clear, specific, and concrete statement of the complaint. Here again, we are simply emphasizing and spelling out what experienced physicians have long known:

> Even in this age of medical technology it is well to remember the words of the nineteenth-century French clinician Laennec, who would tell his assistants and students, "Listen, listen to your patient, he is giving you the diagnosis" (Niederland, 1983, p.163).

Information about the complaint should include *what* is being complained of, *who* is mainly concerned (as the examples indicated, this may not be the patient but another member of the family), and just *how* the matter complained of is a source of concern. This latter may not be self-evident, and inquiring about it may clarify just why the patient has come for treatment. In addition, particularly when a symptom that is complained about is of some duration, it is useful to ask what led the patient to come in *at this particular time.* Often, general questions such as, "Why have you come to see me?" elicit only vague or general answers, which need to be followed up more specifically. In this case the information gained by inquiry about the particular precipitating circumstances may be especially helpful in revealing a hidden agenda: for instance, that the patient has come under duress from another family member rather than voluntarily, or that the problem complained about is not the patient's main concern but only, so to speak, his ticket of admission.

Ordinarily, this information about the presenting complaint can best be obtained by direct inquiry. Asking for examples is often helpful in getting specific and concrete information from patients and family members. If a patient is stressing what appears to be a minor problem, asking how it affects the person's daily life may bring an enlightening answer. For example, a man might present to his physician what appears to be a minor lesion of the penis-a small abrasion or heat rash. Yet his concern seems excessive and he does not seem relieved when told "It's not much of anything." If, then asked how this condition concerns him, he might respond with, "I just wondered if I had contracted something more serious." If asked, "Serious, how?", he might elaborate that he thought it could be a venereal disease and that for some time he has suspected his wife of having an affair but has been afraid to confront her directly about it. Thus, the lesion itself was not a significant problem for him, but what it represented to him was. The most likely difficulties involve patients who give vague, general, or tangential responses. Persistence in posing specific questions will often resolve these problems; the main danger is to assume one understands what the complaint is when it has not been clearly stated by the patient. While this may appear to save time, it is likely to lead to more time lost in fruitless or misdirected effort.

2. It is important to determine what the patient and family members are doing that may be promoting the persistence of the problem or hindering its resolution. In family therapy most complaints are reducible to problems of troublesome but persistent behavior, and the therapist accordingly is looking for other behavior which may be provoking the problem behavior, or at least blocking change. Such unwitting "maintenance" behaviors may also be significant in family practice. For example, the wife of a patient who complains of anxiety and apprehension may be telling him there is nothing to be worried about. The patient takes this as an indication that she doesn't understand the seriousness of his situation, and this understandably increases his anxiety.

In addition, in family practice this kind of information may be very relevant in two further respects. Patient or family actions may strongly influence evaluation of the importance or significance of any given symptom or problem, and as noted, either under or over-concern will present special obstacles to satisfactory resolution of a complaint. Last, but by no means least, even when a problem is strictly a physiological one, what the patient and family members are doing may obstruct effective cooperation with the medical plan of treatment. For instance, a man can have diagnosed diabetes and the maintenance regimen requires some considerable restriction in his diet, restrictions which he himself is willing to undertake. However, his wife, in her over-concern about his welfare and her desire to "make it easier for him to do without forbidden foods," puts the whole family on a restricted diet. Now he is under additional pressure, feeling that the whole family is suffering because of his health needs. He may try to resolve that problem by making light of his condition and departing from his own diet to show his wife that such restrictions are not all that necessary. In such a case, the physician can, with little time and effort, avoid diabetic incidents by talking with his wife and letting her know she can be of most help to her husband by not rearranging the whole family's routines and diet; but the physician is not likely to get very far if he concentrates only on the patient, constantly urging him to be "more careful."

Our experience is that the best approach toward obtaining information about possible problem-maintaining behaviors is to ask the patient, and any closely involved family members, *what they have been doing in their attempts to resolve or ameliorate the problem complained about.* This is a logical and legitimate inquiry, since it is explicitly aimed at behavior closely related to the matter of primary concern. As with the investigation of the complaint itself, this inquiry should be direct and aim for clear, specific, and concrete answers: "*Who* is doing *what* (including *saying* what) in attempting to improve this situation?" We have found that when this kind of information is reviewed with a deliberately critical eye-in effect, asking oneself, "Can I see any way in which these actions might actually be making matters worse?"—it will often appear that the "solutions" of the patient or family members may well be part of the problem: The iron pills mother gave to strengthen a child she saw as being in weak health led directly to his symptoms. Though this may seem ironic, it should be no great surprise. People often try to cope with problems themselves before they seek professional help and, with the best of intentions, they may (especially when anxiously concerned) readily make errors in judging the nature of a problem, in inappropriately applying conventional "remedies," and so on.

Even if it should turn out that the patient's and family members' attempted remedies are not maintaining the problem in any discernible way, such an inquiry lays a foundation for any necessary further exploration, and at the same time the information gathered helps clarify just how the patient and family view the problem-its nature, origin, severity, and so on. Getting their views can be critically important in obtaining their cooperation in treatment, as we will discuss later, *especially* when these differ, perhaps widely, from the physician's own view.

3. Resolution of a presenting complaint, in either family therapy or family medical practice, may occur in either of two general ways. First, of course, the problem complained about may be modified or eliminated, thus removing the grounds for the complaint. Sometimes, a problem may be resolved by simple reassurance and a little time for this to take effect, analogous to prescribing "Take two aspirins and call me in the morning" when a patient is anxious about a minor or self-limiting physical problem. However, if such simple measures do not work, it is not wise to repeat or increase them, any more than it is to continue to treat an infection with the same antibiotic that has already been tried without positive results.

In those difficult problems with no discernible physical basis, or which persist after a physical basis has been identified and treated appropriately, it is likely that a behavioral origin exists, probably centered in the patient's or family's ameliorative efforts, as mentioned above. Once such a complaint-reinforcing behavioral pattern has been identified, the crucial change needed is to get the patient—or the family member—to cease doing it; the problem ordinarily will then self-extinguish. However, *it is usually necessary to get the person to do something else instead,* because it is difficult or impossible simply to stop doing something. That is, one must substitute a new behavior that is incompatible with the one that functioned to reinforce the symptom. This might be some action that is useful or healthy in itself; for example, an anxious or depressed patient might be induced to substitute long walks for sitting and ruminating about his condition. But this is not essential; engaging the patient in any action which blocks the undesirable behavior will be useful, even if the new activity is otherwise trivial or neutral.

A complaint may also be resolved by *changing the patient's, or the family's, interpretation and evaluation of the problem situation.* This does not mean that the family therapist or family physician should attempt false reassurance where a serious behavioral or medical problem exists. But there are two common situations where promotion of some reevaluation of the original complaint is pertinent or even essential. First, the patient, or the family, may be "making a federal case" out of a basically normal situation, as when parents become too anxious and concerned about a child's minor misbehaviors, or someone becomes hypochondriacally fixated on interpreting ordinary bodily sensations as symptoms of some serious disease. Then reassurance is the main treatment required, though providing it effectively may require indirect or strategic means.

Second, there are also complaints for which the best or only answer lies in getting those concerned to view a difficulty as being something that must be accepted and lived with, because it cannot be changed. For example, a moderate degree of memory loss upon aging need not in itself seriously affect an individual's ability to function adequately. But if the individual or family members become alarmed about this as a sign of "senility," and become anxiously involved in efforts to improve things, this creates a *pressure to perform better* that is likely to worsen primary functioning further. The situation can be similar in physical disabilities of almost any degree—after a certain point further efforts at treatment may not only be useless but also interfere with the patient's getting on with life to whatever extent is still possible.

In some cases both reevaluation and behavioral change may be needed to resolve a complaint.

4. In many cases, one matter is crucial throughout treatment: How can the physician gain the cooperation of the patient and family members? This may be critical even in obtaining needed information at the very outset of a case; certainly it will be critical when it comes to promoting any needed actions and changes effectively. With "good patients" and sensibly cooperative families there is no problem; they will recognize the physician's knowledge and authority, and accordingly will give information, take medication, institute actions, and accept reassurances as he or she directly proposes. But not all are good patients and families. Many can be balky and non-compliant; some are over-

compliant ("Twice the prescribed dose must be twice as good") or over-dependent on the physician to do everything while they sit by passively. And, unless the way is well-prepared, almost anyone may be difficult when it is proposed that a person should change a view or an action that is firmly, even though mistakenly, held as *the* right and proper stance toward a problem.

We suggest—similar to our emphasis on getting clear what the patient's complaint is—that the key to gaining effective cooperation in difficult cases lies in recognizing the patient's, and the family members,' own views of the problem and treatment, and then utilizing these in the service of whatever changes are essential for effective treatment. It is only natural that the patient and family members will have views of the problem that differ, often considerably, from the physician's professional observations. First, they are laymen, and second, they are personally involved and therefore highly subjective. The second factor can at most be moderated, not basically changed. Even for the first, while certain explanations are appropriate and essential, in a busy medical practice (as in brief family therapy, only more so) there is no time to reeducate the clients to any level of understanding comparable to the physician's own; indeed, to attempt this is likely to provoke dissatisfaction and resistance by patients and family members who are attached to their views and mainly want to get on with resolving their complaint as soon as possible. Also, no general reeducation is necessary. All that is essential is to obtain cooperation and compliance with those views and actions which the physician recognizes as critical in resolving the problem, and these usually will be quite limited and specific-such things as adherence to a treatment regime, reevaluation of the seriousness of a complaint, changing certain particular behaviors that reinforce the problem.

In our experience, *patients go along with treatment best if the physician does not argue with patient views.* Where a change of stance or action is essential, this principle can still be utilized. There are two main types of such situations. First, a patient or family member may have some recognition that an action is needed but show hesitation about getting on with it. If the person persists in such ambivalence after the physician has explained the need for action, it usually is of no help to do so again and again. Instead, it may be very helpful for the physician openly to side with the patient's doubts for a while: "On second thought, I must agree with you that while the operation is likely to be helpful, there always is some risk, so think it over carefully before deciding." Such an overt recognition and joining with the patient's doubts and fears can be reassuring and thus lead to the desired action.

As suggested earlier, however, in many difficult cases the task is greater. It involves getting the patient to stop doing something that is reinforcing the problem, or even to do the opposite, although he or she mistakenly views the present behavior as necessary or essential. Here the same principle of avoiding argument and resistance by accepting and joining with the patient's views as much as possible is applied by "reframing" the situation so as to lead to a change of stance and behavior. That is, the point in question is presented at first in terms of the patient's own views and language—the way he sees and describes it; but then, rather than arguing with his view, something is added—further information or an added perspective—so that the situation's significance and implications for action, in the patient's own eyes, are now altered or even reversed. A patient might stubbornly balk at following some medical regimen (medications, rest, dietary changes, etc.), insisting that he has never been one to pamper himself. Since his frame of reference is that he wants to be regarded as a strong person, the physician can use that frame of reference to gain his cooperation. He can frame the situation as one "that requires extraordinary strength of character and self-discipline to make the sacrifices necessary to take care of one's body when it has special needs."

A number of the above points are illustrated in the following example: A post-myocardial infarction patient reveals that he has not followed his physician's advice to eat more sensibly and "Don't push yourself." The patient explains he has never been used to "pampering" himself nor seen himself as a "cripple." Besides, he has a lot to do taking care of the animals on his ranch, and their care and welfare come first. The physician is not likely to gain his cooperation by reiterating that he has a serious and potentially lethal medical condition and he has got to take it easy. The patient will hear that as a warning he has to see himself as crippled and no longer up to his former robustness. Instead, the physician can appeal to a value which *is* important to the patient—that he is a caretaker of others. Thus, he can analogize the patient's body with the animals he tends:

> Look, you respect your horse. He'll take you wherever you want him to go, and all day if necessary. When you bring him back to the corral, you're not going to throw him some moldy hay. And when he's put in a good day's work for you, you're not going to take him out again all sweaty and wet. I'm only asking that you have the same respect for your body. It needs taking care of, too, and only you can do it. Do you have enough self-discipline to do that?

Of course, similar analogies can be used for patients in many other kinds of work in which a high value is placed on respect for and judicious care of the tools and materials of one's trade.

## Application of the Approach to the Examples

In the preceding sections, we have described briefly the main foci and principles of our approach as it can apply in family practice, but this sort of statement is a long way from the detailed realities of daily practice. To move at least a step closer, we will conclude by returning to our original examples and outlining how these cases might be handled in actual practice.

In the case of the hypertensive patient, assuming that the medication is appropriate for his type of hypertension and that serial blood pressure readings show a sustained elevation, further information must be gathered. To start with, the patient needs to be asked to describe more explicitly *exactly how* he is "faithfully" following the physician's directives. It is always possible that the patient interprets that what he is doing is what the physician asked, when in reality it is a significant departure. If he is actually following instructions, then other kinds of information need to be elicited-mainly, is he experiencing some significant psychosocial stress at home and/or in his job? Depending on the information elicited, the appropriate treatment might not be a matter of changing dosages or medications but, rather, one of getting the patient to adhere more accurately to the regimen, or one of helping him to deal more effectively with the stresses he is facing. Detailed questioning often yields unexpected information.

With the mother who complains that her overweight child is not eating enough, the key is for the physician to recognize that her complaint, though misguided, is a reflection of her basic concern to ensure her child's health and welfare. To argue with her that, if anything, the child needs to lose weight is not likely to be successful, since this appears contrary to her own values and perceptions. It may even be taken as an accusation of failure on her part to be a duly protective mother. Instead, she needs to be effectively reassured about her motherhood, so that she can then relax about the child's eating. This can be accomplished if her "protectiveness" is supported, but in a different direction:

> It might be better if he ate more, but after careful examination it seems that the food you give him is remarkably nutritious so that, even though he could be eating more, he is in good health. Thanks to the care you put into the selection and preparation of his food, he is a healthy child. Moreover, every child wishes to have some distinctiveness from other members of the family, and I believe his thin image is important to him for his own individual identity. It may require a sacrifice on your part to allow him to hang on to that identity for as long as he needs it.

If the mother is thus successfully reassured that she is a good mother, and indeed that this involves some sacrifice, she probably will lessen her pressure on the child to eat, and the weight problem will gradually resolve itself.

A general point is also illustrated by this extreme case of over-concern—the more usual situation is one of excessive worry based on scanty evidence, but this mother's concern is so great that it overwhelms and inverts the evidence. In either situation, the discrepancy between the patient's position and the physician's observations is so great that there is a strong tendency simply to state this professional view as a means of clarification and reassurance. The danger is that the patient will not respond reasonably to this but will restate the original concern, perhaps more strongly. If the physician is drawn into reiterating *his* statement, then a covert or overt argument has begun, and this will probably lead to a stalemate unsatisfactory to everyone. If the physician can keep in mind that such excessive concern is itself a prime indicator that the patient is thinking illogically (in this one particular area), he is forewarned to avoid the trap of attempting logical persuasion with an illogical person.

Instead, the physician might test the waters by one, preferably tentative, direct statement of clarification and reassurance. For example, I imagine some people have said that he seems to be eating enough and that his weight looks OK. Have you been told that and, if so, what do you think of that kind of comment?

The physician is not committing himself to that comment, only putting it out to check the mother's commitment to her view. If this does not go well, he can then shift toward meeting the patient's emotional need and concern on the patient's own ground, as the above example illustrates. This will also lay the foundation for cooperation in any medically necessary actions.

Resolving the problem of the child who has been passing black stools depends primarily on adequate inquiry, to discover the mother's concern about "sickliness," and her giving of rather large doses of iron pills, which she had not associated with the symptom. Thus, she is duly alarmed at what appears to her to be a worsening of some mysterious illness. In this case a simple explanation might suffice to reassure her and thus discontinue giving the pills. If not, the "symptom" could be redefined as the body's normal and healthy signaling that it no longer needs the iron pills and that it was fortunate she paid attention to this signal.

The unconcerned husband coming in for a physical is likely to be there under some duress from his concerned wife. Thus, he will not be cooperative since he regards the examination as an unnecessary nuisance. He simply wants to get through with it as fast as possible so that he can pacify his wife-which neglects the fact that she is quite unlikely to be pacified unless he cooperates and takes the examination seriously. The physician is unlikely to succeed by appealing to logic, by saying that the wife may have legitimate reason for concern, or that it is important for everyone, including the husband, at least to have a routine physical. The patient is discounting the need for a physical examination, based on the position that there is nothing really wrong with him and that his wife is therefore silly in her concern and urging; he is very likely to view any such statements as joining with the wife's position, and he will therefore resist them.

However, the physician can increase the chances of cooperation by using the patient's own position. He can frame the examination as a challenge to the husband's own veracity or judgment:

> All right, your wife is concerned and it may well be an unnecessary concern. It may be best that you don't allow yourself to be examined, because you might not want to take any risk that she could be proven right. By not having an exam and not giving me the information I need for the history, you can avoid bringing this issue down to the mat to see just who is right about the state of your health.

The framing here avoids getting involved in the counterproductive argument of "You could be sick"—"No I'm not," and puts it on the implied basis, "Are you a big enough man to put your money where your mouth is?" Then the husband is more likely to cooperate, and the wife is more likely to be satisfied, whatever the specific outcome of the examination.

With the apprehensive young man who keeps insisting on further tests, the first requisite is an adequate inquiry into the complaint and its circumstances, a history taking that includes attention to the interpersonal context in which the symptoms are occurring. This will disclose the pending marriage, whose possible connection with the patient's vague but persistent physical complaints is not hard—for the physician—to see. However, it should be assumed that the patient has some resistance to considering this rather simple connection, or he would have done so already. Therefore, any direct or forceful approach to this possibility is likely only to increase the patient's resistance and further insistence on the physical nature of the problem.

There are two aspects to handling this difficult situation more strategically. First, the physical: The apprehensive young man, insisting on further tests, is not going to be reassured should the physician try to talk him out of these as unnecessary or do them begrudgingly, even should further tests prove negative." It is more likely that the young man will insist on yet other tests, or seek other physicians and go through the same route. The physician stands a better chance of heading off this inappropriate path if, rather than resisting, he himself can suggest a further test and say:

> I would like to do another test. I don't think it is necessary, but I would rather be absolutely sure. I don't expect the test to show anything wrong,

but, as I say, I would prefer to err on the side of overcaution than the other way.

Then, as anticipated, should the test come back "negative," the patient has been prepared for that and the confirmation of the physician's prediction heightens his credibility on his overall judgment of the patient's status. This credibility will be heightened even more, since the physician suggested the test and not the patient. It is possible that in a moderate case of this kind, such action will be sufficient to reduce the patient's concerns to a normal level, or at least enough so that he is able to bring out his underlying anxieties about the marriage.

If not, the physician is still in a more favorable position to initiate some consideration of the interpersonal and psychological aspects of the patient's situation, since he has dealt with the physical side at some length and in a way credible to the patient. This can usually best be accomplished by suggesting that, *in addition* to physical factors, some psychological ones just *might* be relevant to his symptoms, since everything in life has both physical and psychological aspects. Such a phrasing is much easier to go along with than any statement implying, "It's all in your head"; acceptance of this possibility, limited as it appears, opens the door sufficiently to begin whatever discussion of the patient's life situation seems necessary to relieve his anxiety—perhaps just by characterizing it as normal: "Every man is nervous before marriage; it's a very big step." This, in turn, can resolve the demand for more and more physical tests.

In conclusion, we would like to emphasize that, while the approach to observing and dealing with family factors in medical practice discussed here is simple in principle, its application to practice is a different and more complex matter, as indeed the application of principles to the variability and individuality of specific cases always is. On this matter, in a limited space we have only been able to offer some brief illustrative examples; moreover, practice ultimately can only be learned *by* practice. Nevertheless, we hope that this introduction may provide stimulation and guidance toward taking that next step.

## References

Fisch, R., Weakland, J., & Segal, L. (1982). *The tactics of change: Doing therapy briefly.* San Francisco, Jossey-Bass, 1982.

Henao, S. (1982). Personal communication.

Herr, J., & Weakland, J. (1979). *Counseling elders and their families: Practical techniques for applied gerontology.* New York: Springer.

Niederland, W. (1983). Importance of case history. *Psychosomatics, 24,* 163.

Watzlawick, P., Weakland, J, & Fisch, R. (1974). *Change: Principles of problem formation and problem resolution.* New York: Norton.

Weakland, J. H. (1977). "Family Somatics"—A neglected edge. *Family Process, 16,* 263-272.

Weakland, J. H., Fisch, R., Watzlawick, P., & Bodin, A. (1974). Brief therapy: Focused problem resolution. *Family Process, 13,* 141-168.

# CHAPTER 15

# Myths About Brief Therapy;
# Myths of Brief Therapy[1]

## *John Weakland*

Let me explain my title and clarify what I intend to discuss in this chapter. By "myths about brief therapy" I mean myths held—at least for the most part—by people outside the field, not themselves engaged in practicing brief treatment. Correspondingly, by "myths of brief therapy" I mean myths held by people within the field, engaged in practicing some sort of brief therapy. However, although this is a useful distinction for the purpose of organizing a discussion, it should not be taken as always plain or absolute. It will become clear that there are overlaps across this boundary, especially that myths *about* brief therapy may carry over into the practice of brief therapy, and by doing so strongly influence that practice.

I will not attempt to be comprehensive, either in terms of including all myths currently relevant to brief therapy or in terms of a complete examination of any particular myth. Rather, I will select a few major myths and clarify the messages, explicit and implicit, that seem functionally most important, i.e., most influential in defining an attitude or line of action toward the practice of brief treatment.

---

[1] Originally published in J. Zeig & S. Gilligan, (Eds.), (1990). *Brief Therapy: Myths Methods & Metaphors*, NY: Brunner/Mazel, p. 100-107.

## The Nature of Myth

It is first essential to say something about "myths" in general, to make my view and usage of this concept clear. Let me begin with a negative statement, to make plain what I do not mean—that I am departing from perhaps the most common idea of myth. I do not see "myth" as an opposite of "truth," as presenting a fantasy in contrast to describing "reality." Instead, I see myths in general as explanatory schema, as ways of using language to interrelate, order, and make some kind of sense out of some set of observations about nature or life. Both the area of interest and observation and the style and clarity of the language employed in giving some ordered account may vary widely. Yet the basic nature and function of myth making are the same for a primitive tribe's myth of the origin of the world, the scriptures of a world religion, or a scientific theory—even in physics.

To put it bluntly, we cannot state what "truth" or "reality" is, and we will never be able to do so. Many, perhaps most, would view this view with alarm: Where is the firm ground we can stand on? Instead, the greater danger lies in the desperate quest for certainty and the accompanying labeling of myths as truth, or worse, as *the* truth, no matter to what conflicts or impasses this leads. And there is much evidence—from the large scale of history to the small scale of our own work with specific human problems—to support this. This may be one reason why Milton Erickson, though himself a great mythologist—a creator and user of stories and metaphors—was so careful and skeptical about building theory with a capital "T," preferring instead to emphasize the variability of individuals and events and the need to garner specific information on concrete behavior.

On reflection—especially reflection on our own field of problems and treatment—it is rather evident that we do not live by realities, but by *interpretations* of observed events or situations. Even our observations—since we can never attend to everything fully and equally—depend on preconceptions of what is most significant. Even when we evaluate the significance of simple specific behaviors of ourselves and others, interpretation of the meaning of any given behavior may vary widely. One wife may see her husband's frequent late return from work as meaning "He doesn't care for his family," while another sees it as "He cares so much he works extra hard to provide for us." Obviously, interpretation has great consequences for the relationship. And finally, to compound the uncertainty of observation and interpretation, the language we use, not only for interpretation but even for description, necessarily is symbolic and therefore always basically metaphorical.

If one can never have certainty, but only interpretations, what is the point of examining myths in general, and myths concerning brief therapy in particular? The point is this: As humanly constructed interpretive schema (whether constructed deliberately or arising out of social interaction), myths embody and summarize ways of looking at things; they show how people have been accustomed to viewing a certain area of experience. And beyond this, there is the other side of the coin. In another example of Bateson's dictum that every communication is both a report and a command (Ruesch & Bateson, 1951, pp.179-180), any such explanatory schema also proposes how the matter in question *should* be understood and responded to, and this is a directive outlining proper thought and action. Thus, in a fundamental sense myths are like maps; they shape and order our understanding of a given territory and guide our steps in traversing it, or avoiding it, and as ancient geographical maps often warned, "Beyond this point be monsters." Similarly, maps may be judged pragmatically, by their usefulness in helping us get to where we aim to go. In the present case of brief therapy, the territory of concern is that of human problems. The means of travel consists of therapeutic concepts and associated practices, and the goal is effective and efficient (and *therefore* brief) resolution of such problems. On this basis, it is useful to examine some major views concerning brief therapy, so that we may see as plainly as possible the basic views of the territory these myths project, what they propose to lead us toward or away from, and the means of locomotion they recommend.

Two different aspects need to be considered in evaluating and comparing myths as maps. First, there is what in a general sense may be called the content of the myth. This is the major concern of the present necessarily limited examination. The main lines of what the myth says must be summarized as clearly and concisely as possible, to get an overview and not be lost in details. But this is not all. Myths often imply much more than they state explicitly, and since implicit content is usually more general, it is likely to be of great importance in determining broad orientations and the interpretation of more specific details. For maps of psychotherapy, for example, unstated differences in underlying general premises may be critical for understanding differences in approach. Therefore, it is important to make the implicit content of myths explicit, as well as this can be done.

Second, there is what may be called the form of myths of psychotherapy. This includes the breadth of the area covered, the economy of the myth's account of this, its completeness, and its clarity. That is, while attempting to formulate a clear and succinct account of the content of any myth, it is important always to remember that its raw original state also strongly affects its functional usefulness as a map. For example, some myths of psychotherapy are stated in such vague terms that their guidance is ambiguous. Others, while more specific and explicit, are too complex and detailed to follow surely. And especially, where basic premises are left implicit and taken for granted, the voyager may be led in critical directions without recognizing this influence.

## Myths about Brief Therapy

Quite naturally and expectably, the most important myths *about* brief therapy—the outside view—come from the proponents of conventional long-term psychodynamic treatment, as the traditionally predominant model of psychotherapy. It is striking, however, that in several important respects these traditional psychodynamic views are quite similar to popular lay views about problems and their resolution, and even to some basic tenets of physiological / biochemical views. There has been so much elaboration, branching, and dispute in a hundred years of myth development about psychotherapy that one easily could get lost in the details, yet it seems possible to discern a few fundamental lines of general significance.

Probably the most important and common characteristic of this viewpoint is that brief therapy—if seen as possible at all—is seen as inherently and drastically *limited* in scope. Two major kinds of limitations, different in kind yet basically related, are posited:

1. Brief therapy is necessarily limited to minor goals or symptomatic treatment, but cannot effect any significant or fundamental change. It is supportive treatment, either as a stopgap or as a second-best measure when real long-term therapy is not available. This may be because either the patient or the helping system is limited in time or money, or the patient is seen as too limited in psychological resources for "real" therapy. The possibility of similar limitation of the professional is seldom considered, though a case can be made that brief therapy requires greater skill than long-term treatment.

2. Brief therapy may be of value in, and should be limited to, minor problems, but "obviously" is inappropriate for major ones. (This ranking or distinction of "major" and "minor" problems again seems to be a matter largely taken for granted as self-evident, rather than being seen as a basic and complex issue needing much thought and clarification.)

It is unclear why such a widespread and powerful view of brief therapy as very limited exists and persists, beyond the obvious fact that for 100 years now a heavy investment in the practice and teaching of this view has been made. Yet two critical underlying premises seem implicit, if seldom explicit. Both lead toward supporting the necessity of long-term treatment, although in a fundamental respect they are different, even opposite conceptions. But this, of course, would not be the first instance of incompatible arguments being used to support the same position.

First, there is perhaps the most basic tenet of conventional psychiatric thinking: If a person behaves in ways that are strange enough and persistent enough to bring him or her under professional psychiatric scrutiny, the cause lies in some significant personal deficit—a pathology—within that individual, and the stranger or more resistant the behavior, the greater or deeper the presumed pathology. At the broadest level, this view is shared by those who see the presumed deficit in experiential terms, in terms of psychological makeup, or in physiological/biochemical terms. Whatever the specific cause ascribed to the presumed deficit, it is plain that in this view, at best there is much work to be done to repair, or compensate for, the deficit. This is a possible, and certainly a popular, interpretation of strange and unusual behavior, but it is not the only possible interpretation, or even the only one advocated in the course of human history.

The other line of thinking is more humanistic, even implicitly verging on an interactional view, but no less pessimistic about any possible brief resolution of problems involving human behavior. This is the view—and here again the professional and the layman stand on similar ground—that human life and behavior are inherently and necessarily complex. The obvious corollary is that if someone is behaving in strange and self-defeating ways, it will take a lot of time, thought, and effort to understand such behavior, and probably much more to alter it—if this is possible at all.

Perhaps this is so. But before accepting this as a given and thus accepting only major coping or remedial measures as relevant to human problems, two possible alternative views should be recognized:

First, there is the possibility that we humans make complex problems out of originally rather simple, if difficult, situations. Although we habitually assume that serious problems must have correspondingly large and weighty causes, this is not necessarily so, for at least two reasons. First, what is a large or serious problem is not a given or an absolute, but again a matter of our interpretation, the same also holds for "complexity" itself. In parts of sub-Saharan Africa, for example, syphilis is so common that it is not considered a "problem," only a fact of normal life. Second, now that we have some understanding of cybernetics, it is increasingly apparent that through positive feedback, repetitive error in handling a difficulty—"more of the same"—can readily and rapidly lead to the escalation of an originally minor and simple difficulty into a major problem (Watzlawick, et al., 1974). And this problem may appear different from the original difficulty not only in *scope* (quantitatively) but also in *shape* (qualitatively).

Another, alternative view is that the complexity we discern is, at least in large part, an interpretive illusion. Such an illusion can occur as a consequence of our failure to gather or attend to data that would simplify the picture; or of habits of interpreting the data we have in terms of complexity rather than seeking simpler (and perhaps more useful, if apparently less profound) interpretations; or both. An analogy makes this point clearer: In almost any good detective story, the mystery involved appears both complex and obscure, until at the end the detective reveals the true clarity and simplicity of the matter. Perhaps this analogy seems too trivial and unrealistic, even though much of the literature basic in establishing the psychodynamic approach, including especially the work of Freud himself, approaches the mysteries of "mental illness" and its treatment much like a problem of crime detection.

If this example still seems inadequate or inappropriate, however, consider the case of the organization and dynamics of planetary movements. As long as the Ptolemaic view of an earth- entered universe was held, the more the data that were gathered, the more complex was the explanation necessary to make some order and sense of them. But once people shifted to a Copernican viewpoint, taking the sun as central rather than the earth, the apparent complexity became relatively quite simple.

While it is not a necessary part of the present argument, it is certainly possible to suggest that there are plausible reasons why we might become involved in making or interpreting things as more complex than necessary. To mention just two: This saves us from rethinking accepted premises, which is always a difficult and painful task; and if human problems are seen as complex, everyone involved is, to a corresponding extent, absolved from responsibility for resolving them.

## Myths of Brief Therapy

Brief therapy, in any modern form, is a quite recent development. Moreover its adherents tend to be clinicians, more concerned with practical results than with theory. For both these reasons, the mythology of brief therapy is relatively scanty up to the present; however, we can at least examine what exists.

Since brief therapy is the "new kid on the block," probably there is already more mythology about brief therapy deriving from psychodynamic sources than from those who have moved toward brief treatment as a basically new approach to treatment. The latter may have some advantages in relative freedom from limiting preconceptions, but the former certainly have the advantage of numbers, prestige, and weight of tradition. The guiding myth of brief psychodynamic therapy may be characterized quite simply and briefly as "less of the same." That is, although practice may involve more activity and intensity, the basic views involved in this approach to brief treatment seem essentially the same as those described earlier for conventional long-term therapy: a postulate of brief treatment as basically limited in scope, evidenced by selectivity as to patients accepted for treatment, and based on similar underlying premises about pathology and the complexity of human problems. Much of this is neatly summarized in Gustafson's (1986) book *The Complex Secret of Brief Psychotherapy*; indeed, the title alone offers much of the essence of this myth. This is not to say that the development of this approach to brief treatment is not an important step forward. It is; yet it also seems clearly a step constrained and limited by unquestioning acceptance of the most basic features of the prior conventional assumptions.

Alternative visions of and approaches to, brief therapy instead are based, more or less explicitly, on an interactional view of human problems rather than an individual—pathology view. These approaches largely derive from family therapy, as the primary locus and exponent of a basically interactional view of behavior.

Probably the most extreme view is the one that, I think, can with reasonable fairness be categorized as a strictly technical or procedural view: "Don't confuse me with theory; let's just get clear what interventions a therapist should make, in what situations, in order to solve interactional problems." Although such a characterization often seems intended as a caricature or a putdown of brief treatment, there is potentially more to it than this. Beyond those eager but naive therapists who at workshops demand, "Give me a paradox for this case situation," there are experienced and serious therapists whose focus is mainly on techniques for promoting change. To a significant extent, this again was true of Milton Erickson himself. Although neglect of general principles and a guiding framework may have accompanying limitations or drawbacks, the corresponding freedom from limiting presuppositions as to how things "really are" may also keep open the door to finding useful new practices, which may eventually give rise to useful new conceptions of problems and their resolution. Sometimes theoretical ideas lead to useful innovations in practice, but often it goes the other way.

An intermediate position is taken by some brief therapists, including Haley, Madanes, Papp, and Silverstein, whose basic views are closely related to mainstream myths of family therapy, but who attempt to work briefly by active, and often creative, techniques of intervention. One could, perhaps, see them as the family therapy analogs of the psychodynamic brief therapists, and a similar question arises: How much may these therapists, again unwittingly, be constrained by their unquestioning acceptance of certain premises of conventional family therapy, for example, that a symptom must have an important function, or that a specific problem must reflect an underlying pathology in the family system?

Finally, another myth is that to make progress toward doing therapy briefly, effectively, and over the widest possible range of problems, we must make a fresh start: in effect, to construct a new myth, a new view of problems and their resolution that is minimally constrained by past myths. On this view, both practice and thought basically should be exploratory. I see the work of my colleagues and myself at the Brief Therapy Center of MRI (Fisch et al., 1982; Watzlawick et al., 1974; Weakland et al., 1974) and that of Steve de Shazer and his colleagues in Milwaukee (de Shazer, 1985, 1988)—among others—as exemplifying this view. Of course, no view or myth is perfect and without its accompanying difficulties or defects. To take this sort of view, in any field and especially in a clinically related one, means that one knowingly risks criticism and subjects both oneself and one's clients to certain chances in the present, in the hope of improving matters in both the immediate and more distant future. Clearly, and especially in the present social and professional climate, a more conservative approach is the safer course to follow.

## References

de Shazer, S. (1985). *Keys to Solution in Brief Therapy*. New York: Norton.

de Shazer, S. (1988). *Clues: Investigating Solutions in Brief Therapy*. New York: Norton.

Fisch, R., Weakland, J., & Segal, L. (1982). *The Tactics of Change*. San Francisco: Jossey-Bass.

Gustafson, J. P. (1986). *The Complex Secret of Brief Psychotherapy*. New York: Norton.

Ruesch, J., & Bateson, G. (1951). *Communication: The Social Matrix of Psychiatry*. New York: Norton.

Watzlawick, P., Weakland, J., & Fisch, R. (1974). *Change: Principles of Problem Formation and Problem Resolution*. New York: Norton.

Weakland, J., Fisch, R., Watzlawick, P., & Bodin, A. (1974). Brief therapy: Focused problem resolution. *Family Process*, 13, 141-168.

# CHAPTER 16

# Basic Elements in Brief Therapies[1]

## Richard Fisch

Changes in psychiatry, psychotherapy, and counseling may sometimes stem from events having nothing to do, intrinsically, with those fields. For example, the need to return soldiers to the battlefront quickly during World War I and, more so, in World War II, led to the use of rapid "front-line" techniques avoiding the use of longer term therapy. "Scientific" justification for these shortcuts was made acceptable by redefining incapacitated soldiers as suffering from "shell shock" (World War I) or "battle fatigue" (World War II), rather than from the more pessimistic diagnoses of neurotic or psychotic conditions. Currently, changes in health care delivery and the influence of insurance companies has led to a rekindled interest in and use of "brief psychotherapy." If one were to take a historic perspective, one might see that, throughout the history of humankind, "therapy" was *always* brief, however brutal or mystical or naive we might regard methods used by different tribes, societies, or cultures; for example, trepanning by Neanderthal tribes, ordeals during classic periods in Rome and Greece, shamanistic rituals, voodoo ceremonies, hypnosis, to name a few. "Therapy" was brief until the advent of psychoanalytic concepts and practices near the turn of this century. "Therapy" changed from a *doing* modality in which the change-agent (oracle, shaman, mesmerist, etc.) either *did* something to the troubled/troublesome person and/or had the person *do* something, to an insight or *understanding* modality, one which re-

[1] Originally published in M. Hoyt (Ed.), (1994). *Constructive Therapies.* New York: Guilford Press.

quired a stylized conversation, mostly one-sided. The "patient" was required to be more active in the conversation, therapist more passive, often meta-communicating about the "patient's" comments. Such a modality inherently required a lengthier and more frequent contact between patient and therapist but was "scientifically" justified by the "discovered" findings of such things as "the unconscious" and the role of "unconscious conflict," among, others. Without a historic perspective, one is likely to believe that long-term therapy is the benchmark against which all other therapies are to be measured; that briefer methods are the newcomers often regarded as naïve and superficial, ignoring the fundamental "discoveries" of psychoanalytic/psychodynamic approaches. To give the reader an idea of the pervasiveness of this tradition, many therapists who do not regard themselves as following psychoanalytic concepts nevertheless believe that the presented symptom or complaint serves some *needed* function for the individual or family, a need that the patient or family members need to understand.

Shifting from history to the present, the increased interest in and development of briefer methods has led to a burgeoning of different schools. Some of the earliest are psycho- dynamically oriented approaches, such as those propounded by Alexander and French (1946), Malan (1963), and Sifneos, (1972), but these, for the most part, are more focalized uses of psychoanalytic theory and practice, and differ qualitatively from more recent methods such as those developed by Milton Erickson (Rossi, 1980), Jay Haley (1963, 1977), the Mental Research Institute's Brief Therapy Center (Fisch, Weakland, & Segal, 1982; Watzlawick, Weakland, & Fisch, 1974; Weakland & Fisch, 1992; Weakland, Fisch, Watzlawick, & Bodin, 1974) solution-focused therapy (de Shazer, 1985; O'Hanlon & Weiner-Davis, 1989), and White's narrative method (White & Epston, 1990). In this chapter, I suggest some common denominators among those latter approaches, factors that are unrelated or relatively unrelated to their underlying rationales, their models. Subsequently, I present sequences of an initial session held at the MRI Brief Therapy Center, which illustrates those basic features. This effort is not a comparative study of the different schools but rather a "formula" for making therapy shorter, more efficient, and, likely, more effective. In order for a therapist to utilize such elements, she or he will need some "scientific" or "theoretical" justification, and these are provided by the different schools or approaches.

## Narrowing the Data Base

In general, the greater one's data base, the longer therapy will take, and, conversely, the narrower the data base the shorter the therapy. "Psychotherapy" is primarily a verbal exchange. The therapist asks questions to elicit information and, at some point or points, makes some comments to the client with the intended or unintended effect of influencing the client in some way. (Some therapists say they don't influence their clients; that change occurs through some mysterious transformation presumed to have welled up inside the client. But if a therapist says anything at all, he or she will unavoidably influence-the client; otherwise why be in the room?) The more areas of information sought by the therapist (e.g., childhood experiences, relationships with people not directly involved in the problem, nonverbal communication), the longer will be the verbal interchange with the client, and this length will be compounded since the client's responses to that data will, in turn, be regarded as further necessary data and so on.

How can the data base be narrowed? (It might be useful to keep in mind that the question can be posed conversely; i.e., how can the data base be expanded so as to lengthen treatment?) Therapies that regard the problem as occurring in the present and that regard present or current data as principal will have eliminated a considerable body of data referable to the past, certainly the distant past. If, within that time frame, the therapist concentrates on eliciting descriptive data ("What did you do when. . . ?" and, "And then, what did you say?"), rather than explanatory and inferential data ("Is it that he's lazy?" or, "Why do you feel it's necessary to . . . ?"), it can save considerable time.

Explanatory data lends itself to expansion and connections with other ideas while descriptive data is limited to the event being described; for the most part, it has a logical endpoint. For instance, descriptive data might be: "Mainly, he doesn't do his homework. We'll come home and he's usually sitting watching TV, and if we remind him to do his homework he just glowers at us and goes to his room and turns on his radio." Explanatory data might sound more like the following: "I think his school problem stems from his low self-esteem. That started as far back as when he was a toddler. My husband would get so angry with him if he stumbled and knocked something over. You know, John was never a patient man and, throughout Billy's growing up, john was always criticizing him, never giving him credit for anything. Like the time Billy was building a car model. . . . I think he was eight or ten at the time; anyhow, be got a little glue on the workbench and, when John saw that, he flew into a rage. It was so sad to see Billy's look of defeat. But John had been treated the same way when he was a boy. His father was an alcoholic and when John would come home..."

Therapists will also narrow their data base if they regard the client's complaint as the only problem to be resolved rather than believe that other departures from "normalcy" also need changing, even if the client is not complaining about them. This latter effort is consistent with those models that have a normative feature, that is, where the therapist operates on the idea that there is an important and objective standard of human behavior such as mental health or healthy family functioning." Thus, while the client brings in one problem, the therapist can "identify" another or a number of others, which "require" working on, and which; naturally, expand the data base considerably. Focusing only on the client's *complaint* can avoid this elaboration of therapy. It can narrow the data base even further, in obtaining a statement of the complaint, the therapist asks the client to prioritize among elements in the problem. This kind of effort reduces time in therapy by focalizing the problem to be resolved. This is distinct from the traditions of therapy that tend to broaden out the complaint and, thereby, increase the data base. "What is the *main* thing your spouse does that gets to you?" will focus the client more than, "You say you've experienced this trouble before. When was the first time and how often has it occurred since? Would you say there's a pattern here that needs understanding?"

## Intrapsychic Versus Interactional Concepts

A therapist can lengthen treatment by viewing the complained about behavior as stemming from some quirk or pathology lying within the individual. This is not so easy to avoid. It happens to be a major feature of traditional and extant therapies and is the common parlance of everyday conversation and exchange of ideas. ("Oh, he's just an angry person"; "We're developing a profile of the typical abuser"; "You know those car salesmen are just crooks"; "I'm a real procrastinator"). It can prolong treatment in a number of ways: First of all, since it usually involves some concept of pathology, the individual/ family members and therapist are faced with implicit pessimism when attempting to change a fixed or pervasive condition, such as the difference between looking at the way a person *is* versus what a person is *doing* in a given context in interaction with others. The task of change will be regarded as more intimidating with the former view and expectations of change—how much and how quickly—will be significantly diminished. Secondly, an individualistic (intrapsychic, monadic) viewpoint limits the therapist's and the client's options for changing a complained about state of affairs; since it is presumed that the problem lies within the individual, it follows, logically, that the person must be the main focus of therapy regardless of whether that individual shows sufficient interest in changing or not. (In the latter case, therapists will usually explain non-change in therapy as resulting from the client's "resistance" or "denial.") Metaphorically, the therapist is limited to banging at the same door and cannot exercise the option of looking for and possibly entering other doors. Finally, data referable to a person's inside" are "softer" than descriptive data. The latter is more easily obtainable when addressing an interactional sequence.

"Well, he walks in the door and asks me 'is supper ready yet?' When I tell him 'No, it's gonna take a little more time,' he blows his cork. 'What the hell do you do all day you can't get a simple meal ready when I'm hungry'!"

*Versus*

"As soon as he gets home, he's hostile, although I'm not sure if he's been that way at work. Anyhow, he can't even say hello; he just gets extremely impatient, and he wants to put me down, especially those things I do to take care of him. Nothing I say will satisfy him, and he just seems to lose control like I've seen him do with friends when we've visited them."

As mentioned before, it can save a lot of time in therapy to use descriptive data. It is tangible and succinct. Intrapersonal data, instead, is abstract, explanatory, and can more easily be elaborated upon.

## Influencing Change: Task Orientation Versus Insight Orientation

Whether it is acknowledged or not, the therapist cannot *not* influence the client. For that matter, it is the function of the therapist to influence the client, presumably in ways that benefit the client, otherwise, why have the therapist present or, at least, why say anything at all? One dimension of therapy-time-will be influenced by the therapist's view of whether the major modality for benefit derives from the performance of some kind of task or from the attainment of insight. (I am using "insight" interchangeably with "understanding," "awareness," or "discovery.")

A task orientation will significantly reduce the amount of time needed in therapy. First of all, the fact that the therapist anticipates that the client will eventually *do* something in relation to his or her complaint automatically circumscribes the areas of information sought; for example, it is not relevant to expend much, if any, time asking about the client's early years. Secondly, further time is saved since preparing a client for a task tends to limit discussion on some, perhaps much, previously gained information. That is, there tends to be a paring down or sorting out of data to information having more and more relevance for the formulation of a task or suggestion. Finally, an action tends toward closure, either of the therapy or some step or phase of it. The client does something, and if it results in resolution of the complaint or a step in the right direction, termination of therapy is soon to follow. In contrast, "insight" directed therapy tends towards expansion; "awarenesses" are built on "awarenesses." (This in addition to the time-consuming task of the client learning the therapist's "language"—*proper* "awareness"—and with minimal and implicit cues from the therapist, since "awareness" is presumed to arise "spontaneously".) For example, in the various psychoanalytic approaches, it goes beyond coincidence that classical Freudian analysands will develop Freudian insights, Horneyian analysands Horneyian insights, Jungian analysands Jungian insights, and so forth; yet, it is likely that neither analysand nor analyst are aware of those means, which influence such outcomes. Task-oriented therapists may differ in their methods of inducing action by the client, principally by utilizing explicit directives or by implication or, sometimes, both. While these are stylistic or tactical differences among the different "schools" of brief therapies, they have in common an intention of getting the client to take some action different from those actions formerly taken in the struggle with the problem.

## Goal Orientation: Knowing When to Stop Therapy

How long or short therapy is also depends on whether the therapist knows when to stop. It may seem trite to say, but if one has no idea of when something is done one runs the risk of going on interminably. Therapy, therefore, can be briefer if the therapist has some rather clear idea of what needs to occur to mark an endpoint of therapy. The lack of such clear indicators is a feature of a number of models, for example, the psychoanalytic schools, the progenitors of "long-term therapy." It can also be a feature of approaches not particularly characterized as "long term." For example, psychiatrists utilizing an organic/medical model may deem certain criteria as clear indicators for *starting* medications but have less specific criteria for when to *stop;* thus, medications intended for temporary use may be used for years. A frequent dilemma for both the psychiatrist and the patient is that, if the patient is doing well, will stopping the medication bring a relapse? Either the patient or psychiatrist or both may be too uneasy to take the risk. One "solution" to this dilemma is to define a number of problems as "metabolic" or "genetic" flaws, thus justifying lifelong medication.

In summary, then, stylistic, tactical, and/or theoretical differences may be found among most brief therapies, but they are likely to share some basic features. While it is not a complete description of such similarities the preponderance of features of these therapies are a marked narrowing of the data base, utilizing interactional rather than monadic concepts, emphasizing a task orientation, and formulating definable goals of therapy. The following is a composite transcript of an initial session from the MRI Brief Therapy Center, which illustrates these features.

The transcript is the first session with a 35-year-old woman whose husband was seen alone in the first session of the case. He was 37 years old and described his problem as a "block." He had been out of work in his profession for almost a year and said that he was having trouble doing those tasks required for employment, such as, completing a resume, contacting potential employers for interviews, and seeking help from friends for other leads. It is customary for us to see the spouse, to determine if the spouse is also a complainant. (I am using "complainant" to define a person who indicates a clear interest in overcoming or resolving the complaint and who views the therapist as a necessary resource in accomplishing that goal. In that sense, it differs from the common usage of an individual who simply registers a complaint.) This was all the more likely since the husband, Robert, had described his wife, Janet, as very upset about his failure to proceed with job seeking. Her upset compounded the problem since he felt pressured by her, as well as guilty over his failure to get on with the necessary tasks. This state of affairs left a pervasive air of tension in their relationship. From his description, it seemed likely she was a complainant, but we also wanted to assess if she might be the better focus for changing a counterproductive loop. It is difficult to make an absolute assessment of who, in an interaction, is the better focus. Some features that can be used are the degree of expressed discomfort about the problem, responding to questions with appropriate information, and following the therapist's suggestions or directives, among others. The "loop" in this case was the husband's putting off tasks to which the wife responded by pressuring him and to which he responded by further inaction, etc. What follows, then, is the second session, the first one with Janet.

**Therapist:** Let me start off this way: Imagine that I haven't seen Robert, I don't know anything about him, and you are coming in here because of some concern you have about him or some problem you are encountering with him. I'm starting off as if it's fresh and, so if I can assume that either or both are the case; that you have some concern I would then start with: Okay, what's the problem or concern you have?

As in any focalized therapy, an initial session will start right away with some form of, "What's the problem?" Since I had seen Janet's husband first and she had come in at my request, asking her about the problem required some introductory comments. It can also save a lot of time to inform a client that he or she should not make assumptions that the therapist has some relevant prior information ("I'm starting fresh").

**Janet:** My concern is that I see him immobilized, and I guess the most obvious proof of that is that he was *laid off the 1st of April* and hasn't, in my assessment, *hasn't really looked for a job since* then. And I think what brought me to a point of crisis was that I saw that no matter what I was doing, no matter what I could think of to do, it didn't seem like I was able to *help* *him* and that I didn't see him asking anyone else for help. But on a consistent basis what happens is he gets so *demoralized,* actually *immobilized.* It's almost like in *panic* or in *fear* that he doesn't do any of the things that I suspect he's capable of doing.

I have italicized some of Janet's wording to highlight what I call "the client's position." Her phrasing rather clearly indicates that she is not angry with him but feels sorry for him, sees him as having good intentions but being limited in his efforts, and, logically, she sees her involvement in his problem as one of helper rather than victim. It is a useful time-saving aspect of therapy to pay attention to the client's position, since it will help the therapist from making potentially stalemating comments and, more so, to aid in framing suggestions concordant with the client's "reality."

**Therapist:** What would be some thing, or things that he really could do?

**Janet:** See, I'm in a little bit of a quandary. When we met, I knew that he was having some problem with his studies. It was clear to me, although he wasn't admitting it, that he wasn't going to classes regularly, and he ended up dropping out of the program. So, the quandary is, I don't know what job he should be looking for. However, it is important to have at least some sort of resume. You need to look through the paper and network with people and ask them if they know of any jobs anywhere. You have to call people and go to interviews. Those are the sort of practical things that I can see, and I want to be supportive of that, but it seems to me that those basic rules you have to do even if you are uncomfortable, and he hasn't been doing that. The issue of the resume has been an issue since the first week in May and he's made promises to me over and over: "I'll have it by this week and I'll show it to these people"— and I don't think he has a resume. I find myself thinking: "What are you doing hooked up with this guy? Are we going to be able to have the life together that we wanted to?" Then my concerns get more future oriented.

**Therapist:** It will be very helpful to us to know what doesn't work, and so in terms of what you've done or said in your efforts to try to get him moving, what doesn't work?

With this particular client, little time was needed to obtain a clear picture of her complaint; she responded to questions as asked, rather than going off on tangents and, for the most part, gave clear, concrete examples, which quickly clarified material. Thus, it allowed the therapist to seek information earlier regarding her attempts at resolving the problem, what we refer to as the client's "attempted solution." For our form of doing therapy expeditiously, this feature is the single most strategic factor in our model, since information about the client's attempts provide the guideline of what is to be a *different* effort for the client to make. Clarity about this can save considerable time, since it avoids the potential of misdirection in the therapy, which may result from simply asking the client, "What would be different?" Too often, the client will equate a variant of his or her customary effort as different, in the same way a person talking to another who speaks little English may try to make himself clear by saying the same thing, only louder. A very frequent error made by clients, which illustrates this point, is when they equate keeping silent as the extreme opposite of their previous statements: "Well, when I wasn't getting anywhere telling him why he needed to stop drinking, I went completely the other way; I ignored him."

**Janet:** It doesn't work to let myself get to the point where what I do is explode or bitch and nag. That doesn't work, in contrast for instance when I . . .

**Therapist:** When you explode, bitch, or nag, what kind of thing would you say, what would you be saying?

**Janet:** Well . . . it's more the tone of voice.

**Therapist:** Because when you explode, bitch, or nag, you've got to say something—although I know it would have certain decibel levels.

When reporting an event or sequence of interaction, clients will often use "shorthand," that is, a vague summary of what is being said or done. However, this is not usable information and can be misleading, since it leaves it to the therapist's imagination or interpretation what actually occurred. To save time, it is characteristic for us to ask the client for verbatim dialogue. While tonality and other paralinguistic should not be ignored, as a general rule, the content (wording) of a message is more indicative of the thrust of that message.

**Janet:** "You never do this thing . . ."

**Therapist:** Yeah, I'm not asking for a success story—otherwise you wouldn't be here.

**Janet:** Probably saying the same thing over and over again: "I can't count on you"—bringing up, bringing up all the times before—and, "You know, you haven't helped me pay the bills this time, and all these days in the last week you haven't helped me clean up the kitchen and blah, blah, blah, blah," bringing in everything including the kitchen sink, the whole complaint. That doesn't work. It also does not work to just . . . this has been the thing that's been difficult for me; it does not work to just leave him alone. There are times when I just get fed up and I think: "Okay, I'm just going to let him stew." That's one way I explained it, or, "I'm just going to give him a break." I find that that doesn't help, either, that I need to be present. Just because I'm uncomfortable, it doesn't work to be invisible myself, to pull away.

**Therapist:** Say nothing?

**Janet:** So that's the underside of it-that clearly hasn't worked.

As referred to before, this is a common but erroneous assumption made by clients that "giving up" or becoming silent constitutes a difference from what they had been doing before.

**Therapist:** It may not be important right now, but you're implying that if you were going to do anything differently, in the hope that it would be more effective, it would require your saying something, not just like ignoring . . . Anyway, what else have you . . . ?

Since a major element in shortening therapy is planning to help the client *do* something different, it enhances efficiency by preparing the client for the idea that different action will be expected. Here, the therapist is "planting" such an expectation.

**Janet:** Let's say, and he's made this a few times, he'd make the agreement of, "Okay, in these seven days this week I promise to do this every day: Make three phone calls, or work on my resume for half an hour, or go to the job place, and every day I will report to you in the evening about what I've done." That's one way that he's attempted to manage this.

**Therapist:** Will he volunteer that kind of proposal, or would it be something he would come up with at your suggestion, or . . .

**Janet:** I don't think I've ever suggested that. But he's come up with it in the context of talking with other people about what might help and having me be the helper here. But anyway, that is one thing we've tried. He doesn't report it— he may report for a day or two and then it becomes my responsibility, and I'm not, I don't think I'm really so invested in it, I don't think it's going to work in the first place, and so maybe I don't even ask him about it. I'm not sure we've given it a fair trial, but for me that hasn't worked.

**Therapist:** Okay. But the proposal, as I understand it, is, "Okay, every day I will report to you as to what I've done or accomplished with some particular effort . . . ." When he proposes that, what do you say anyway, by the way?

**Janet:** I say, "Okay, okay, how are you going to do it?" I try to get clear about when is it you're going to report to me, what is it that you are going to say, what are you agreeing to do.

Here again, is an illustration of the time-saving effect of getting exact dialogue. Janet's comments just before "I don't think I'm really so invested in it . . . and so maybe I don't ask him about it" implies she takes a more passive or less effortful approach to Robert's proposal. However, when describing actual and specific dialogue, this picture is reversed and confirms her "attempted solution," that of being a taskmaster and urger.

**Therapist:** Okay. And you're saying that what has happened in practice is that for a day or two he might say: "Okay. Here's what I've done today," et cetera . . . but then on the third day or so he doesn't and you don't pursue it?

**Janet:** No, I have sometimes. If I ask him, often what it is that something didn't work out: Either he didn't do what he'd said he was going to do, or he tried to do it and it didn't work. He was discouraged. He might have read the paper for five hours in the morning rather than going out and doing what he said he was going to do. And so he's disappointed in himself and doesn't want to admit it, and when we talk about it, something happens around that that we both get despairing - so that I don't find myself being very peppy: "Well, you know, just go for it tomorrow."

**Therapist:** Again, just so it might save time, could I take it then that the things you've done are the things that everybody else has done like your sister and brother-in-law. They all fit under the general rubric of, "Robert, you can and must make a more effective effort," which didn't work, and everything else would be, in a sense, a variation of that.

Quite often, time can be saved by alerting the client early in therapy to the main direction he or she needs to avoid, what might be called avoiding the main theme or thrust of their attempted (albeit unsuccessful or counterproductive) solution. This helps to serve the client as a guideline for determining what action(s) will be *different.*

**Janet:** Is that what we've been trying to do?

**Therapist:** Yes. That is, it's being put in different ways, angrily, threateningly, *and* coaxingly but my understanding is, they're all different ways of saying, "Come on, get with it," when one sort of boils it down, and that, with Robert, doesn't work. And, let me shift gears again a little bit. You said you've been very frustrated about the situation, and I gather you've been asking yourself: "Why does he just sit there?" That is, you said he's immobilized. You commented that it seems to be, by way of explanation to yourself, you know, some purpose? I guess mainly what I'm asking you is, what's your own guess, and I'm not marking papers, I don't have any answer to that, but what is your best guess as to why he is not making an effort you think he's quite capable of making?

Janet: My guess is that he's *scared,* that he has a dream of doing important recognized work, that maybe would make him famous, that certainly would have him be powerful, that he's *afraid* he's not going to be able to do that. I see more of a problem being that he's a man and his wife is supporting him. I think that's a big deal, that for him shows up as "this shouldn't be happening," and there's no way around it.

Therapy can be lengthened, if not undermined altogether, if the client flatly rejects a suggestion or task that might have helped them out of their stalemated problem. This danger can be avoided if the therapist takes the trouble to frame the suggestion in a way (wording) that is consistent with the client's frame of reference, the client's "language," or, as we have labeled it, the client's "position." Here, the therapist is checking on Janet's "position" vis-a-vis the problem with Robert. As can be seen from her reply, it confirms the earlier indication that she feels sorry for Robert— that he is willing but unable, rather than he is able but unwilling-and this position lends itself to framing any suggestion as one of "helping" him (as opposed, for instance, to confronting him, or getting even with him).

Therapist: Okay, but to whatever degree you're saying that just inherently in the situation "I'm in a one-up position, not only financially, economically," but also you're, I would assume, reasonably satisfied with the kind of work you're doing. So he's way down, so to speak, in both respects: He's not working, but he, you know, imagines what he would like and what's expected financially— same thing— he can't stand working even now. Let me think out loud as if I were you: "Looking back on the things I've been saying, mostly saying to Robert, is what adds up to 'Robert, you've got to get your act together. You can and you must make a more concerted effort in finding a job.' So that's what I've been doing and that's not working. So if I were going to do anything different, what would be different?"

Having received sufficient information regarding Janet's complaint, her attempt at solution, and her "position," the therapist now moves on to address the task of helping Janet with *doing* something— something different.

Janet: What would I do?

Therapist: What would you do or say, so it wouldn't be just a variation on the same old theme? That doesn't work. Second thing I'd like you to give thought to is: Okay, if whatever you would be doing, certainly what Robert would be doing by himself, if either or both of those things were appropriately effective, what would be a very first sign where you could say, "By God, it's not big, it's nothing startling, but it sure as hell is different: that immobility is starting to loosen up."

Since the session is closing, the therapist wants to accomplish several things: summarize the direction therapy needs to go, end on an *implicitly* optimistic note, and convey to the client that active participation in the therapy will be expected of her. This last is conveyed through "homework" in this case, thinking actively about the questions being raised and indicating it will be part of her participation next time. As for optimism, it is always conveyed on the implicit, not the explicit, level, and here it is suggested via the question, "How will you know you are *succeeding?*"

## Summary

I have suggested that there are some few features of psychotherapy that can influence the length and efficiency of therapy and that these features cut across lines of different models or approaches. While these features are few in number, they are fundamental and can make a strategic difference in the time spent in therapy. I have not presented these features in any tightly organized way, and they vary in their relative specificity; for example, narrowing the data base is rather general, while utilizing a task orientation is much more specific. However, while they are elements commonly found in current brief therapies, each approach will have its own emphases, different criteria for terminating therapy, different tasks for therapist activity, and different vocabularies for the same or similar techniques utilized by other approaches.

One word of caution, however, while the elements I have described are few and, I believe, simply put, they are difficult to implement in clinical practice. They are not technical guidelines for therapy; rather, they are *outcomes* of a *conceptual shift* from "long-term" therapeutic approaches. For example, narrowing the data base depends on what the therapist regards as minimally necessary features in his or her conceptual framework. There does seem to be an attraction for complexity. Developments in psychoanalysis afford an example. Analysis in Freud's time might be as brief as six months or a year. Subsequent "generations" of analysts, however, "found" more and more "necessary" features, which required increased work in therapy and today an analysis of three to seven years is not unusual. There is no reason to believe that "brief" therapies will be an exception to this trend.

## Acknowledgements

I wish to express my deep appreciation to Barbara Anger-Diaz, PhD, for her immeasurable help in preparing this chapter. Without it, this chapter might not have been written.

## References

Alexander, F, & French, T. M. (1946). *Psychoanalytic Therapy.* New York: Ronald Press. de Shazer, S. (1985). *Keys to Solution in Brief Therapy.* New York: Norton.

Fisch, R., Weakland,J. H., & Segal, L. *(1982).The Tactics of Change: Doing Therapy Briefly.* San Francisco:Jossey-Bass.

Haley, J. (1963). *Strategies of Psychotherapy.* New York: Grune & Stratton.

Haley, J. (1977). *Problem-Solving Therapy.* San Francisco:Jossey-Bass.

Malan, D. (1963). *A Study of Brief Psychotherapy.* New York: Plenum.

Q'Hanlon, W., & Weiner-Davis, H. (1989). *In Search of Solutions: A New Direction in Psychotherapy.* New York: Norton.

Rossi, E. (Ed.). (1980). *The Collected Papers of Milton Erickson* (Vols. 1-4). New York: Irvington.

Sifneos, P. (1972). *Short-Term Psychotherapy and Emotional Crisis.* Cambridge, MA: Harvard University Press.

Watzlawick, P., Weakland,J. H., & Fisch, R. (1974). *Change: Principles of Problem Formation and Problem Resolution.* NY: Norton.

Weakland, J. H., & Fisch, R. (1992). Brieftherapy-MRI style. In S. Budman, M. Hoyt, & S. Friedman (Eds.), *The First Session in Brief Therapy* (pp. 306-323). NY: Guilford.

Weakland, J. H., Fisch, R., Watzlawick, P., & Bodin, A. H. (1974). Brief therapy: Focused problem resolution. *Family Process,* 13, 141-168.

White, M., & Epston, D. (1990). *Narrative Means to Therapeutic Ends.* NY: Norton.

# CHAPTER 17

# "To Thine Own Self Be True..." Ethical Issues in Strategic Therapy[1]

*Richard Fisch*

As the title suggests and this chapter will clarify, strategic therapy calls for a shift in emphasis in ethical thinking from "honesty" as a primary value toward personal responsibility as a primary value. Ethical issues apply to every form of therapy—as well as any other transaction between people—but are more salient in strategic therapies, which emphasize the deliberate use of influence by the therapist. Ethical issues regarding therapist influence often are less controversial in traditional insight-oriented approaches since the goal of therapy is principally to aid the client to become aware of, or gain insight into, those factors and events defined as relevant by the particular therapist. In strategic therapies, however, higher regard is given to directives, tasks, and "homework." When therapists are faced with getting clients to *do* things, they are faced with the task of persuasion. With the increasing interest in, and use of, strategic therapies, it is to be expected that more questions of ethical practice will come to the fore.

One example of this concern is Phillip Booth's (1988) presentation at the 1986 Erickson Congress. Another recent, although less extensive treatment of the subject, is a book by O'Hanlon and Wilk (1987). A chapter on ethics has

[1] Originally published in J. Zeig, (Ed.), (1985). *Ericksonian Psychotherapy, Vol.* I: *Structures.* NY: Brunner/Mazel.

been written by Zeig (1986). Most of my comments address Booth's work because of the extensive and thorough way in which ethical issues are addressed and the way he relates them *to* theoretical and philosophical considerations. Booth argued:

> ... for the removal of "trickiness" and manipulativeness from strategic therapy and *to* rewrite the techniques of strategic therapy according to commonsense and with nontechnical terms. (p. 39)

The intent of this chapter is *to* argue that, 1. manipulation is unavoidable in *any* therapy—and in any human interaction; 2. the measure of its benefit or detriment is in the outcome of therapy; and 3. the choice is not whether or not one is manipulative but whether or not one acknowledges to oneself the use of manipulation.

The title of this chapter alludes to this concept. In the course of developing these positions, I will examine the premises on which Booth bases his contentions as well as his own form of persuasion in presenting premises and conclusions *to* the reader.

## Booth's Position

Booth appropriately begins his argument with a discussion of philosophical questions regarding reality since they have a direct bearing on ethics. In his criticism of the concept of reality as a subjective matter, he misses the point that this is an alternative *viewpoint to* the traditional *view* of reality as an objective matter. This misunderstanding is apparent in his statement: "if the *existence* of an objective real world is *undermined,* the *objective facts* of that world *become* ephemeral" (p. 43, italics added).

He incorrectly interprets constructivist thought as denying what is factually there. He does not grasp that objective reality and subjective reality are two different *beliefs.* Based on this misunderstanding, Booth proceeds to his ethical position: *"Regard for the facts* is thereby *undermined* and therapists can tell lies with philosophical *impunity"* (p. 43). He warms to this theme with some fervor: "The most serious *attack* on the *obligation to* tell the truth when conducting therapy stems from an *attack* on the notion of 'reality'" (p. 43, italics added).

Constructivism is not a heresy as Booth's language implies. Rather, in offering an opposing view of reality, constructivism opens up an alternative ethical base: Ethical and responsible therapy involves working with the client's reality (frame-of-reference, world-view, etc.), rather than requiring clients to accept the therapist's reality. In failing to understand constructivist thought, Booth incorrectly attributes to strategic thera-pists an adversarial position vis-a

-vis their clients ... placing emphasis on truth and honesty. This requires adopting a non-adversarial view of therapy contrary to that which is often promoted by strategic therapists. (p. 40)

Equating "truth and honesty" with being non-adversarial is a questionable position. Webster (1975) defines adversary as: "A person who opposes or fights against another, opponent, enemy." One certainly can oppose, honestly and/or truthfully. More important, attributing an adversarial position to strategic therapists disqualifies the fact that in strategic therapies, as in all therapies, the goal of the therapist and client is mutual; that is, resolution of the client's problem. Booth negates the fact that the therapist uses knowing manipulation to achieve a *mutual* goal. Ironically, the strategic therapist, in deliberately using manipulation, is more likely than the traditional therapist to respect the client's "reality," seeing it as a *different* reality than his or her own rather than an incorrect or "unhealthy" reality. To enhance the client's motivation to accept a suggestion or task, the strategic therapist utilizes the client's "reality" and may say things when explaining the suggestion that do not reflect the therapist's own "reality."

This is anything but "adversarial." Adversarial positions are more likely to arise when the therapist believes the client's reality is "mistaken" or "dysfunctional" and sets about to correct that "reality" in accordance with his own perceptions:

"But Joanne, might you be misperceiving your husband's intentions?" "Oh, no, I know him too well. He does that with everyone." "He does that with everyone? You had said that he doesn't do that with your son." "Oh, that's different. Brian knows how to get around him."

I'm sure this kind of dialogue must sound familiar to every therapist. It is an example of the frustrating and counterproductive arguing that often occurs when one tries to get the client to "look at reality." As a handy face-saving device, therapists always can say that they are being realistic and that it is only the client who is being oppositional.

After disqualifying proposals about alternative views of reality, Booth shifts by implying that philosophy about reality isn't that important anyhow, that the central ethical point is the *intention* of the therapist in what he says to the client. Although objective truth is elusive, we *can know* when we are being truthful, that is, saying what we believe or what we know to be the case and we *can know* when we are lying or fabricating, that is, saying, with the intention to deceive, things that we do not believe or what we know not to be the case. This is a "central-argument that is quite separate from any philosophical argument about the attainability of objective truth. (p. 45, italics in the original)

I agree that "intention" is the central ethical point, but not in the way that

Booth uses the concept: What Booth intends and what strategic therapists intend are quite different. Strategic therapists, for the most part, believe that what the therapist says—regardless of the "honest" intention of that statement—will have some influence on the client. This, after all, is a basic tenet of interactional thought; that is, you cannot not influence. Thus, if the client responds in an unfavorable way, whether or not the statement was "truthful" or "deceptive," the strategic therapist is more likely to reexamine the presented message since, technically and ethically, the therapist accepts responsibility for influencing the client. Booth, it would appear, divests himself of such responsibility since an untoward reaction by the client is secondary in order for therapists to maintain a good feeling about their "honest" intentions or attitudes. He puts this quite succinctly:

> My comments on this (i.e. a therapist taking a "one-down" position), as well as on other tactics, relate to the therapist's attitude and not simply to some pragmatic criterion of whether that attitude "works" or not. The fact that it *does* is not the justification for it. The attitude cannot be reduced to a tactic or technique. (p. 49)

This obscures to *whom* it is or is not justification and implies that there is some objective standard of ethical practice and that a therapist is either ethical or not. Booth does not leave room for the idea that therapists may have *different* ethics, differences that depend on how the therapist sees his moral obligation to this client. (There are *some* ethical rules that apply to every therapist; e.g., no sex with clients.) Thus, since Booth puts higher priority on "honesty" than on results, for him to say something he does not believe would be unethical. Conversely, for the strategic therapist, results take higher priority than saying what one believes. Thus, to be truthful for the sake of truthfulness, without regard for the outcome on the patient, would be unethical. It is self-deception to believe that if a client responds adversely to a "truthful" utterance, the therapist has not influenced that client in unfortunate ways.

Booth then seems to backtrack from his moral position of truthfulness for the sake of truthfulness by invoking the concept of "unconscious:" However, a client's unconscious mind is not fooled by promises made on this basis [referring to a therapist falsely reassuring the client] any more than it is fooled by some affected protestation that the situation is even worse than he or she thought, such as this tactic suggests. (p. 49)

This puts the matter back to the pragmatic necessity of honesty since it would seem to work better than deception-based, of course, on the premise of an "unconscious," which screens for insincere intent. (Wouldn't it be nice if such reliable mechanisms were operating within the voter during political campaigns!)

Since my central point is that manipulation, wittingly or unwittingly used, is an inherent element in human communication, the choice for therapists, ethically speaking, is whether or not to acknowledge to themselves that they are being manipulative. Booth illustrates this self-deception rather clearly:

> For example, to parents who have been extremely worried about their child who has now shown improvement I often say they should give some thought to what they are going to talk about together now. If I want to emphasize the point by hinting that even their sexual relationship may have been neglected because of their preoccupation with their child, I might ask them what they are now going to talk about *when they go to bed at night* (p. 51).

But why hint? Why not say it forthrightly, as he so strongly defends? I agree with his manipulation in this clinical vignette but he is not saying what he believes, and further, he is saying something he does not believe, namely, that the couple needs to have a conversation when they go to bed. By his own definition, this is "manipulative" and dishonest and therefore unethical. It requires self-deception to deny he is being manipulative. Similarly, O'Hanlon and Wilk (1987), who are close colleagues of Booth, are caught in a self-deceptive snare. They too take the "dishonest" strategic therapist to task:

> Again unlike—some other therapists, many of whom we respect greatly, we do not try to be tricky in doing therapy. We are not trying to do something to our clients. Our therapy would not be unsuccessful if our clients found out what we are doing. Our stance is emphatically *not* one of "tricking clients out of their problems." Trickiness is, in our view, disrespectful to the clients and totally unnecessary to carrying out effective psychotherapy (p. 162).

Yet, earlier they described some of their techniques:

> Frequently we "summarize" what a client has been saying ("Let me see if I understand this so far ..."), but in the summarizing we introduce a significant twist of some kind. Our summary includes all the significant facts of the client's story so far and perhaps some aspects of the story the client has woven around those facts, but introduces a twist in the story—to which we do not draw attention, but which is offered merely as part of the summing up. We get the client to "ratify" our summary and to add "anything we've missed" and then we proceed on the basis of

the version of the story so far represented in our summary (p. 126).

And:

A related operation involves interrupting a client after he has said something significant but before he can go on to specify what he thinks the
significance of his statement is or what the implications are for solving
the problem. We interrupt to agree with the point made and sometimes
stress its importance or insightfulness, and go on to attach a rather different significance to it from which the client might have intended to
attach to it. Again, I agree that these manipulations can be constructive
in helping clients resolve their problems. However, my point is that it
requires self-deception to state, that one is above trickiness and then
describe techniques that are clearly "tricky" (pp. 126-127).

In espousing his particular ethical position, Booth recognizes that he is potentially caught in a dilemma because of his high regard for Milton Erickson's
work. Not only does much of current strategic therapy stem from Erickson's
work, but Erickson himself used manipulation with patients and was quite
open about it. In addressing this troublesome disparity between Erickson's ma-
nipulativeness and his own commitment to "honesty," Booth most clearly illustrates what I would call self-deceptive reframing. He begins by acknowledging
that Erickson used deception in his work: "It is clear, then, that Erickson was
not always honest in what he said to his clients" (p. 46). Having had to make
that admission, he quickly proceeds to what can only be described as semantic
sleight of hand: "But how manipulative was he?" (p. 46), implying that, somehow, it's not quite unethical to be dishonest as long as one isn't manipulative.

However, even this reframing isn't enough since Erickson boldly acknowledged that he was manipulative. This requires another act of self-
deception: "It can be argued, however, that there were aspects of Erickson's
work that distinguish it from the questionable manipulation of much modern
strategic therapy" (pp. 47-48). Booth develops this theme first by acknowledging that strategic therapists, in their use of manipulation, adhere to the moral
position that it be used to aid in the resolution of the client's problem and not
self-servingly. Yet, after the acknowledgment, he discounts it:

This is fine, but the problem with this view is that, thus defined, manipulation loses its ordinary meaning: The use of under-handed or unethical
means to influence people. The illusion is thereby created that manipulation in the bad sense, that of abusing people, does not exist. (p. 47)

The "illusion" appears to be Booth's creation since he had just cited and acknowledged the principal ethical position of strategic therapists that manipulation can and should be used humanely and responsibly, rather than malignantly; to do otherwise is to manipulate without accepting personal responsibility for the manipulation and its outcome.

Booth then arrives at his major argument for distinguishing between Erickson's manipulation and that of strategic therapists. Since, technically, it is difficult for him to differentiate between what Erickson did with or said to patients versus that of strategic therapists, he does an interesting reframe: "There is a profound difference of attitude between Erickson and the strategic approaches referred to at the beginning of this chapter" (p. 48).

He summarizes the "wrong" attitude as one he defines as "adversarial" and, further, identifies a "good" or "bad" attitude by the *explanation* the therapist gives for her interventions, not by the intervention itself or its outcome. Thus, for example, if the therapist explains technical manipulations with the vocabulary of "strategy," "tactics," "games," "maneuverability," and so forth, then one has an "adversarial" attitude and is therefore unethical. Conversely, if the explanation is given in benign terms, "helping the client," "leaving the client to choose," "understanding the client's needs," and so forth, then, one has the "correct," "non-adversarial" attitude and is, therefore, ethical.

Booth, of course, does not question whether therapists, including Erickson, believe their explanations. For example, since Erickson's explanations most often were responses to his being questioned, was he answering "truthfully" or manipulating the interviewer? Similarly, are many strategic therapists uncomfortable with their "caringness" and compassion for their clients and thus lying when they claim to believe they are really being tough-minded and calculating?

I deduce from all of Booth's arguments that his central measure of whether a therapist is being ethical or not depends, in the final analysis, not on *what* the therapist says, or its effect on the client, but on whether or not he can convince others that his statements and intentions are "sincere." While he focused on the authors of *The Tactics of Change* (Fisch, Weakland, & Segal, 1982) as the quintessence of manipulative therapy, he did bestow approval of one of their explanations of a tactical ploy:

> One non-adversarial explanation for this tactic is provided by Fisch, et al. (1982, p. 160) themselves when they say it removes a sense of urgency for the patient—a sense of urgency that has probably been fueling his persistent attempts at "solving" his problem. (p.50)

I suppose the question for Booth is; were the authors of *The Tactics of Change* being sincere?

# References

Booth, P. (1988). Strategic therapy revisited. In J. K. Zeig and S. R Lankton (Eds.), *Developing Ericksonian Therapy: State of the Art*. NY: Brunner/Maze!.

Fisch, R., Weakland, J., & Segal, L. (1982). *The Tactics of Change: Doing Therapy Briefly*. San Francisco, CA: Jossey-Bass.

O'Hanlon, B., & Wilk, J. (1987). *Shifting Contexts: The Generation of Effective Psychotherapy* (pp. 126-127, 160-163). NY: Guilford Press.

Zeig, J. (1986). Ethical issues in Ericksonian hypnosis: Informed consent and training standards. In J. K. Zeig (Ed.), *Ericksonian Psychotherapy, Vol. I: Structures*. NY: Brunner/Mazel.

# CHAPTER 18

# Brief Therapy MRI Style

## *John H. Weakland* and *Richard Fisch*

How one conducts treatment—and evaluates its outcome—depends to a large extent on one's general view of the nature of problems and their resolution. Therefore, any attempt to convey an understanding of the handling of a specific case treated in psychotherapy, in addition to a description (or better, exemplification) of case specifics and their discussion, also must describe the model of therapy within which the therapist is operating, or, at least, believes he or she is operating.

In the present case, this is likely to involve certain difficulties, and we think it may be helpful to start by giving fair warning of these. First, although we have been working on and using this model for more than 20 years at the Brief Therapy Center of the Mental Research Institute, Palo Alto, CA (MRI) (Fisch, Weakland, & Segal, 1982; Watzlawick, Weakland, & Fisch, 1974; Weakland, Fisch, Watzlawick, & Bodin, 1974), and have taught it widely, it is quite different from the psychodynamic approach that is still the prevailing model in psychotherapy generally and probably even in brief treatment. Moreover, it is different in some basic respects even from conventional family therapy, out of which it grew. Second, the model itself (though not necessarily its application) is very brief and simple. Perhaps this should not be a cause of difficulty—indeed, in scientific work generally, theoretical simplicity is considered a highly

[1] Originally published in S. Budman, M. Hoyt, & S. Friedman, (Eds.), (1992). *The First Session in Brief Therapy*, NY, Guilford Publications, p. 306-323.

desirable aim. Yet, it appears that the world of human problems commonly is assumed to be unavoidably complex, so that people have difficulty believing that a simple model could be relevant and effective. We can only report that a number of people who have read our publications and then come to see our actual practice say, with some surprise, "You really do what you say you do!" and that it seems to work.

In common with the general orientation of family therapy, our center views problems as interactional—that is, not as something residing within a particular individual, but as an aspect or a resultant of interaction between individuals in a family or in some other system of social interaction and communication. Consonant with this, we view problems as behavioral in nature—that is, as consisting of some persisting behavior by the identified patient which is stimulated and shaped by behaviors of other persons involved, or sometimes by other behavior of the patient himself. We see problem resolution, accordingly, as requiring behavioral changes by those involved in the system of interaction, and the essential business of the therapist as the promotion of such change, which the members of the system have not been able to accomplish on their own.

We differ from many family therapists, however, in our focus of inquiry and intervention, our means of promoting change, and our goal and evaluation of treatment. In large part, these differences may be seen as related to our pursuing the interactional view of problems further than is commonly done, both in concept and in practice. To start with, we concentrate on the presenting problem and behaviors that are directly related to this, much more than is usual. Correspondingly, not only do we avoid looking behind or beneath the "symptom" as is emphasized in dynamic psychotherapy, we also avoid looking around it broadly as in much of family therapy. Our aim is to narrow, rather than expand, the treatment field.

More broadly, this focus on the presenting complaint has increasingly led us away from the dichotomous conceptual framework of "pathology" versus "normality"—with its implication that there is only one right way for an individual or a family to function. Instead, our view of problems and treatment is essentially complaint based. Likewise, our goal of treatment and the basis of its evaluation are resolution of the original complaint. This, after all, is the basis of entering into therapy in the first place.

Since we also take the concept of interaction more seriously than many do, we believe it is possible to bring about whatever change is needed to resolve a problem in a system through promoting change in any one member, with the expectation that this will, in turn, promote change in other members. The immediate consequence of this view is that instead of seeing all members of a family routinely, we concentrate our treatment attention and effort on whomever seems most concerned to see change happens—not necessarily the identified patient—or the one who possesses the greatest leverage in the system. That is, who we see directly in treatment, as well as the nature of our inquiries and interventions, is a matter of strategic choice.

Now, to be more specific: If one really focuses on behavior, any problem of the kind people bring to therapists may be defined as consisting of, 1. some observable behavior, which 2. is characterized as undesirable (deviant, difficult, distressing, dangerous) either by its performer or by some other concerned person, but which 3. persists despite efforts to alter or get rid of it, therefore 4. the concerned person seeks professional help. Accordingly, our treatment begins by inquiring *who* is doing *what* that is seen as a problem, *who* sees it as a problem, and *how* is this behavior seen as a problem. (We may also inquire, especially with long-standing problems, just what provoked the client to call requesting help at this particular time.) Throughout this inquiry-and in subsequent inquiries equally-our aim is to get as clear and specific a description as possible—who is, observably, doing and saying what. That is, we see the behavior of concern as itself the problem, not as just "the tip of the iceberg," another sign or symptom of some more fundamental inner or deeper state, or even, necessarily, a manifestation of some deep and pervasive disarray in the system of interaction.

On this basis, we next inquire not about the nature of interaction as a whole in the family, but about the behavior most immediately related to the problem behavior, namely, what is being said and done to try to handle (prevent, resolve) the problem by the identified patient and/or any others concerned with it.

Both a general viewpoint and concrete experience underlie this concentration of attention. The interactional view of problems implies a cybernetic rather than a linear concept of causation. Therefore, with this view, it is not the origin of a problem but its persistence that is central for understanding and treatment: What unwitting behaviors function to maintain or reinforce the problem behavior, even though this is defined as undesired or undesirable? Ironically, in our clinical experience it appears over and over that some aspect of people's attempts to control or eliminate the problem—though these attempts are usually well intentioned and seemingly logical ("common sense")—constitutes the reinforcing behavior: "The 'solution' is the problem" (Watzlawick et al., 1974).

In other words, problems consist basically of vicious circles, involving a positive feedback loop between some behavior labeled "wrong" and inappropriate (i.e., ineffective) efforts to get rid of it. Several features of our approach follow from this view. Our general treatment aim is to interrupt the vicious circle maintaining behavior. Accordingly—except in a limited number of cases where the problem behavior can appropriately be redefined as "no problem" or "just one of life's difficulties"—our specific interventions aim primarily at interdicting continuation of the misguided "solution" behavior. Since one cannot just cease any given behavior, such interventions often involve the prescription of some new alternative behavior, but the crucial element remains stopping the performance of the attempted solution. An apparently small change in this respect can be strategic; it may initiate a reversal in the feedback loop, leading to further positive change.

In making such interventions, we do not try to bring about overall revision of the client's intellectual understandings or behavioral patterns. Our concept of a problem is that it is a limited behavioral issue in which someone is "stuck" —although its effects may have spread widely. Our corresponding aim is to help clients get "unstuck" so they can get on with the daily business of life as they see fit. A problem may be solved by behavioral changes—ceasing the attempted solution—or sometimes by a reevaluation of the original focus of complaint as "no problem," just one of life's daily difficulties. In promoting either sort of change expeditiously we "speak the client's language," and avoid argument, as much as possible, although our questions and suggestions imply a behavioral and interactional view of life with a strongly pragmatic orientation. Such interventions mainly involve suggestions for behavioral changes in the real world outside the therapy room. Usually, however, these are not direct prescriptions but depend on reframing the problem situation, avoiding argument, and utilizing the clients' own preexisting ideas about people and problems-speaking the client's "language"—so as to make different problem-handling behavior appear logical and appropriate to them. Since our aim is specific behavioral change rather than intellectual understanding (which may produce no change in actual daily behavior), we do not devote much effort to clarifying and discussing the overall interactional system to those involved. However, behavioral change may lead to new views; also, our mode of inquiry and intervention may promote a pragmatic and behavioral view by implication.

## Case Illustration

The case presented is typical of our work in most respects: It closely follows the model sketched above; the problem is similar to many encountered in our practice; the family is self-referred (although we do get some referrals from physicians or other therapists); and there was no intake procedure beyond filling out a simple demographic information form, since we believe that information gathering is itself a basic aspect of treatment. In one respect, however, this case was not typical, but in a way that helps to underline a major emphasis of our usual procedure. Ordinarily, we would conduct the initial interview with that member of the family we regard as the main complainant. Most often this is the person making the telephone call asking for help. We can confirm this by asking how motivated the other members of the family are: "How eager to come for therapy?" If it is reported that any one or more are "eager," we include them in that first session. In this particular case the caller, the identified patient's mother, said she would be quite glad to come in as soon as possible. Unfortunately, she added that she was about to go away for a 2-week business trip but asked if we would go ahead and see her 19-year-old son about whom she was concerned. She indicated that he was "interested" in coming in, but it seemed to us that his motivation was questionable. Ordinarily, we would have waited until his mother returned from her trip and have seen her first, alone. As it happened, we were about to do a workshop and were counting on this case for a live demonstration of interviewing methods. We therefore decided to go ahead for the sake of the workshop and see the son first, despite our misgivings about his motivation. As it turned out, he was rather passive about his problem—"I get into fights"—and apparently more concerned about his mother's nagging than any consequences stemming from his fighting (e.g., a broken arm).

The identified patient, Bob, had a 21-year-old sister, Jean; his mother was 47 and divorced. In the first session with Bob, he explained that his currently broken arm was actually a re-fracture of a broken arm that had occurred during a previous fight and had not healed sufficiently before this last fight. He also mentioned that he had recently gotten arrested simply by "loudmouthing" police when they came to investigate a complaint about the behavior of some of his friends. He said he himself had not committed any offense, nor was he under investigation, but his verbal abuse and aggression were such that police felt it necessary to take him into custody. His stance throughout this interview confirmed our prior view that he was not a serious "customer" for treatment.

The following interview with his mother, Nancy, was for us, then, the beginning of treatment, and thus we consider it the initial interview since it is more representative of our approach. We have not included, in the transcribed excerpts given here, our usual orienting the client to the features of the Brief Therapy Center such as our audio and videotaping, observation of treatment by other members of the team, the schedule of our follow-up interview, fees, and the like.

## The First Session

**Therapist (Fisch):** What's the problem?

*We want to convey to clients that the counseling will be a problem-solving venture. We usually do this by starting right off with, "What's the problem?"*

*or "What's the trouble that brings you in?"*

**Nancy:** Well, I don't know what the problem is, but the reason he's here is he's angry.

**Therapist:** What I mean by "What's the problem?"—I don't mean anything profound by it and I don't mean the whys and wherefores, but just that, assuming you are coming in because you are concerned about him, my lead question would be, "What reason do you have to be concerned ... what's the trouble?"

*It is not unusual for a client to interpret the question as asking for "why" there is a problem or what the underlying reason is for the problem. In those cases we will explain to indicate we are asking for the client's complaint, that is, what is the behavior she is concerned about.*

**Nancy:** Well, he has been arrested twice. He did nothing wrong except he couldn't control his temper. He really didn't break the law but he kept hassling the policeman. He hassles me all the time. He used to be delightful and fun and laughing. Now I'm with him 2 minutes and I'm ready to scream. He's just angry. He gets into fights. That's not like him. I guess you know he's broken his arm five times now, three of them fighting. He's going to kill somebody or get killed. I ... he's just not a happy kid. He's miserable and he's making me miserable.

**Therapist:** Can you give me an example of that or how would that go?

*As can be seen, Nancy describes the problem in general and vague terms and we need to have the complaint described in specific and tangible terms. The most frequent was we do this is by asking for an example since this tends to direct the response toward descriptive terms.*

**Therapist:** Well, recently where he was fine, and then he starts to change in his behavior?

**Nancy:** Okay. Monday he came home from the hospital and he was fine and we discussed all this and he was so relieved and delighted and he was pleasant and helpful, and we'd laugh, and I said, "Bob, I haven't seen you laugh in so long." Everything was going great. I left for Boston. Tuesday morning and I called in Tuesday night. First thing he says is, "Jean isn't home. She hasn't been around. Nobody's cooked my dinner, nobody's ..." "I said, "Bob, wait a minute. I'm in Boston I can't, I can't do anything about this." And I said, "Talk to your sister," and he knew where she was "and ask her, if you need something, if she could come home. Call me back." This is in

Boston. "Jean won't come home!" "Well, you're mobile; you can take care of your problems and . . ." He called me seven times that night complaining. Finally, I said to him, "Bob, you're out of control again. You're, you're. . . . All this good behavior is gone. You're right back to where you were." And then his sister called me there and said, "Mom, he's calmed down, he's okay now." I . . . but . . . he's 19 and he called me that many times. . . ? And I don't deal with it well. I just think, why can't he appreciate that I can't do this? *(Long pause)*

Therapist: That's in part because the reasonableness doesn't work.

*Usually, after a client has given a sufficiently clear presentation of the complaint, we will ask, "How do you try to deal with it?" In this case, she has included her attempts to deal with Bob's demandingness, and the therapist decided to intervene by reframing her efforts at exhorting Bob to calm down as being "reasonable." Choosing such a reframe has two advantages: (1) it is non-critical of her, and (2) if the client accepts that being "reasonable" doesn't work, she is in a better position to accept a suggestion to handle things in a "nonreasonable" or "unpredictable" (i.e., very different) way.*

Nancy: I always lose. I always give in first. I always back down. I can't deal with the high velocity thing. I've never liked it. I back off ... and he knows that.

*Her response indicates that she has accepted the reframe, at least to the extent of agreeing that her customary attempts don't work.*

Therapist: When you get angry, what kind of thing would you be saying?

*Again, another attempt to have the client be more specific and descriptive.*

Nancy: I would be trying to make him hear what he is saying to me; "Now, Bob, why are reacting like this? Why are you doing this to me?"

Summarizing excerpts from that session, the following information is pertinent to our approach:
1. The mother is the complainant, certainly the principal complainant.
2. Her complaint is that Bob fails to exert restraint on his impulses, resulting in frequent fights and arrests outside the home and infantile demandingness at home.
3. She has attempted to deal with this problem by pointing out his unreasonable stance and exhorting him to modify his demands. In particular, when

she feels it necessary to deny his demand—"No"—she attempts to get him to acknowledge the correctness" of her decision.

We next include an excerpted transcript of the second session with Nancy to illustrate how this information is utilized in the treatment. The reader will see that it takes up where the previous session left off.

## The Second Session

**Therapist:** The way you've tried dealing with Bob normally, is to try to he reasonable?

*This is not intended to elicit information so much as to confirm that the client has still accepted the reframe described in the first session. This is important before going ahead with any other agenda since acceptance can provide for a time-saving shift or step in treatment, the building block, so to speak, for a specific suggestion later. The suggestion will offer an alternative way of dealing with Bob's demandingness, a suggestion that will interdict her more customary and counterproductive method.*

**Nancy:** Uh huh, and I give in a lot. That's also a way of dealing with it.
**Therapist:** Okay, but that's in part because the reasonableness doesn't work. He needs to come to terms...
**Nancy:** Yes. He needs to grow up, and he knows that too.
**Therapist:** Well, he knows and he doesn't know it.
**Nancy:** I think he knows the difference . . . and what it is going to entail.
**Therapist:** And I'm saying that, in particular, I think a good part of your helping him would be avoiding, as much as you can, legitimizing his stuff, his comments when he's coming on abrasively, demanding, being unrealistic about it.

*The therapist is deliberately being general and vague. Previous responses indicate she has accepted the idea that her being "reasonable" doesn't work, the therapist is not certain enough that she is ready to accept a specific suggestion and he is using these general comments to see how she responds to them. We would prefer to make the error of taking unnecessary time- "playing out the line" than risk the alternative error of making specific suggestions too precipitously. That latter error invites the client to discount the suggestion and, thereby, diminish the therapist's credibility. This can cost far more time in treatment.*

Nancy: I do what?

*The client appears to be asking for specific instruction but without indicating her position on the previous remarks. Because of that, the therapist continues with noncommittal statements.*

Therapist: Well, if you are not going to be reasonable, then, I guess, it would be some form or forms of being nonreasonable. It would be any form that, mainly, would convey, without argument, there's no room for discussion on this. This is not a legitimate thing to discuss anymore than what should you pack to go to Mars. That would be in general. Let me show you how tricky it is because to say, "Look, there's no point in discussing this," is to be reasonable.

Nancy: Yes ... "And why can't we discuss it? And just give me three reasons why we can't discuss this."

Therapist: Right.

Nancy: "Well ... because ..." and then I'm into discussing it.

*Here, the client gives a "Yes" response. She indicates she has gotten the therapist's point.*

Therapist: That's right, it's tricky.

Nancy: He's demanding. What do I do then?

Therapist: Well, as I said, it is how to respond to that in a way that delegitimizes his unreasonableness, because it needs to be for his own benefit, in a way that just cuts it short, no discussion, it's not worth discussing and, also, where it doesn't lead to further polemics, that is, doesn't get his back up.

Nancy: That's the problem.

Therapist: I'd say a part of it may depend on your willingness to be a bit arbitrary for his sake, because arbitrariness is a way of cutting short things, like, "Go fight City Hall." I'm not saying to say that but just everyday arbitrariness.

*Despite the client's apparent readiness to take a different tack, the therapist is still being noncommittal and probably unnecessarily cautious.*

Nancy: So I just have to be firm in the ... "I can't handle this, I can't deal, I can't answer your problem; you are going to have to do this. That's it!"

Therapist: Well, it would have to be something that is just unarguable, no point.

Nancy: I haven't found one of those.

Therapist: Well, if you don't mind the onus, since you've said, looking back, there are a number of things I've done, a lot of things I've done that I don't think have been for the best.

Nancy: Of course.

Therapist: Okay. So to that extent, it would be quite true, you could say that you haven't been as good a mother as you would have liked.

Nancy: Uh huh.

Therapist: And that if you don't mind the onus, you might be willing to say "that's wrong." That after talking with me, you've come to realize that you haven't been "as good a mother as I had hoped."

Nancy: And?

Therapist: Period. Then, when he calls and says, "I want you to take care of this," you can say, "No, I won't. If I were a better mother, I would."

*The therapist has finally decided to be more specific judging from the client's attempts to formulate some specific plan. As the reader can see, the therapist hasn't simply come out with, "Here's what to say . . ." but has built a logical sequence of thoughts, each resting on the previous one. This is rather usual for us, since it gives the therapist a chance to back away if the client is not giving "yes" responses at each step. Here, Nancy responds with "Of course." and "Uh huh.")*

*(Long pause)*

Nancy: How interesting! *(Laughs)* This is so good because I would have come at it from the other side: "I am being a good mother now, by not solving all your ..." and I would have gone into this long dissertation making me look okay because I wasn't doing what I *knew* I shouldn't be doing. That's wonderful!

*This is a very encouraging "yes" response. Quite often, when the client is intrigued by a suggestion, one can be fairly certain the client will carry it out. In her final statement, "That's wonderful," the therapist avoids a one-up stance by making a one-down comment, in this case, "Well, keep your fingers crossed." This is intended to imply that the suggestion might not work at all and, therefore, might not be such a brilliant piece of work. Avoiding a one-up stance allows the therapist to take a flexible position regarding a suggestion: it will either work and thus maintain or increase his or her credibility or it won't work, something the therapist will have already entertained and, in that way, protect his credibility. Also, we prefer that the client not feel she is a passive and helpless puppet fortunate enough to have encountered a master puppeteer but is an active participant in the resolution of the problem.*

**Nancy:** Oh, it may not always work, but it certainly ... it will stop him for a while.

## Summary

In all, eight sessions were spent. Bob was seen twice more (one of them a split session with his mother); the rest of the sessions were with Nancy. The sessions with Bob confirmed our initial impression that he was the less strategic person with whom to work. He remained quite passive in his participation. The work with Nancy pursued the strategy begun in the second session with her, mainly to get her to depart from her customary attempts to have Bob accept her "No" by trying to convince him of the legitimacy of that "No." As a way of departing from that, the therapist reinforced the suggestion that she limit the explanation of her "No" to simply reflecting that she was a "bad mother." By the seventh session, she reported she had taken an opportunity to implement this suggestion, with surprisingly gratifying results:

Bob had asked her for the use of her car and she replied she wouldn't do it. When he asked her, "Why not?" she replied that if she were a better mother she would agree but that she wasn't that good a mother. Bob had just shrugged his shoulders, said "Okay," and walked away without any further fuss. By the eighth session she said that there had been some remarkable changes in his mood and his behavior. He seemed happier and had volunteered to help her with the care of the home. As a final comment on his change, she reported on his recent confrontation with police investigating a disturbance. Bob was polite to them and the police wound up apologizing for inconveniencing him.

Since we offer clients 10 sessions in the Brief Therapy Center, the therapist suggested that the remaining 2 sessions be "kept in the bank to be drawn on if and when the need should arise." Nancy was agreeable to this arrangement.

## Follow-Up

As is also our practice, we do a telephone follow-up 3 months after the last appointment. Nancy said that her concern about Bob's violence and his demandingness at home was much less. He had gotten a job as landscaper and had taken up surfing for recreation. There had been no further treatment. Bob reported that he was better able to control his temper and that his relationship with his mother was much improved. He added that he was no longer depressed and that he had not sought any additional treatment.

## Editor's Questions

Q: Your approach can be categorized as "minimalist" in that you focus immediately on creating a small change that will interdict soil aspect of the interactional cycle in which the problem is embedded. The solution-oriented
models have also been described as "minimalist," although they emphasize
"exceptions to the problem" rather than the problem itself. What do you
see as the advantages of one approach over the other?

A: We agree that both our approach and that of de Shazer (198 1988), as the
leader of "solution-focused" therapy, can be considered "minimalistic," not
only in seeking a small initial change that will lead on to more but also in
seeking theoretical simplicity—though it should equally be emphasized that
applying either of these orientations practice may be far from simple. Beyond that we do not see these two approaches as opposed or contradictory.
de Shazer was in contact with and influenced by the work of MRI at least
from 1972, when he came to one of our early brief therapy workshops, and
our approaches have much in common. However, we focus primarily on
attempted solution that do not work and maintain the problem, but with
some attention noting and promoting actions that have worked; de Shazer
and followers, in our view, have the inverse emphasis. The two are comple-
mentary.

Q: On what basis do you make the decision about who in family provides the
greatest leverage for change? What are your criteria for determining who
the "customer" is? By talking initially with one family member on the
phone, aren't you vulnerable to getting skewed perspective on the motivations of other family members?

A: Our primary criterion in deciding whom we will work with in treatment is,
"Who is most concerned to make change in the problem situation?" That
is, who is most ready not only to voice a complaint to take some action
about it. A second criterion may be, "Who has most power to effect
change?" This is most significant in child centered problems; parents have
much more power than a child-although they may not recognize this.

   In initially talking to only one family member, by telephone or in person, there is, of course, a possibility—in fact, a certainty—of getting an
incomplete or biased account of the problem situation. But there are also
several important factors that minimize the likelihood of being seriously
misled. First, our inquiries always focus on getting specific, concrete descriptive information about the problem-who says what, who does what?
Such information is much more reliable than general statements. Second,
we usually inquire whether anyone other than the initial complainant is sig-

nificantly involved in either the occurrence of the problem or attempts to resolve it; if so, we usually arrange to meet with that person or persons also. Finally, accumulating experience in talking, either conjointly or separately, with the various persons involved in a problem leads to the increasing ability to evaluate and interpret the partial accounts of persons seen alone.

Q: In your interview there is no mention of the father. What factors in treatment might have led you to ask about the father's role/involvement, etc., and to consider this person in your treatment planning?

A: We routinely ask clients what help or advice about the problem they may be receiving from anyone else, and if it appears that another person is significantly involved, we will often meet with that person or persons also. In this case, neither the identified patient nor his mother indicated that the divorced father was much involved.

Q: What do you see as some of the advantages of using a "complaint-based" approach in contrast to one that uses a predefined set of diagnostic criteria?

A: To answer this large and basic question fully would require at least another article, but some main points may be reemphasized here. We do not believe that there is only one correct or "normal" way for every individual or every family to think and act. Accordingly, in each case, rather than trying to fit people into a predetermined system of categories, we want to know, as clearly and specifically as possible, what is seen as the main problem by the specific client(s) involved, how this is seen as a problem, and what would be seen as a satisfactory resolution. These are the matters that matter to our clients, and for which they are paying us—as their agents—for professional help.

Q: What do you do when you are left with a client who is not a "customer" (e.g., someone referred to you by the courts)? Do you have some strategies for transforming a "visitor into a "customer"? In what situations would you agree to meet with several family members at once?

A: There are two different situations involving clients who come to treatment under duress. When someone comes because of pressure from a family member (or possibly from a friend), we attempt to see and work with the more concerned other person, as we did in the case presented here. If a client comes under legal duress, this is not usually a feasible course. Then we first take steps to define ourselves as separate from the referring authority, and not necessarily in agreement with its views of the client and the problem. After this, it is possible to inquire if the client himself sees any problem that it might be useful to work on. As a last resort, it may be suggested that there is one evident problem-that the client is under duress from an authority— and ways of handling this might be worth discussing. But unless something the *client* perceives as a problem can be established initially, therapy is apt to be only a futile effort.

Q: When the therapist says, "That's because the reasonableness doesn't work," in response to the mother's question, isn't he presenting a linear formulation (i.e., giving an explanation of *why* something is not working)? How does this fit with the idea that the MRI model is based on a circular (nonlinear) notion of causality?

A: The therapist is not really giving an explanation so much as pointing out, "Here is another example of your attempted solution—reasonableness— not working, not producing the effect you desire." Like most people, clients see causation as linear, and we see it as circular, but we do not think it necessary to teach our clients a new general view. If we can just get them to handle the problem behavior differently in specific ways, there will be different responses, and the vicious circle will be broken.

Q: The intervention is a clever and useful one. Did you think about, and reject, other alternative interventions? Could you tell us what they were and why you chose not to use them? In a similar vein, is it often a matter of trial and error to come up with the "right" intervention, which really ends up working? Are there particular principles or guidelines you use to find or develop such an intervention?

A: In this particular case, we did not entertain any different intervention with the mother. It seemed clear enough that she needed to depart from attempting to have her son acknowledge the legitimacy of her "No," and from experience with similar cases, this can often be done most quickly and easily by having the parent take the position of a bad parent." How we motivate the particular parent to adopt that depends on the individual parent. In this case, as in many cases, we will first try by labeling their attempts as "being reasonable with someone who is being unreasonable." In this case it was sufficient so we did not need to look further. In many cases, there is some trial and error, but these different options and trials mainly have to do with finding ways of *motivating* the client to take an action or of designing appropriate actions depending on acceptability to the client, opportunity for implementing them, convenience, and the like. We do not think in terms of "the right" intervention; there are usually many ways of achieving the same goal—the interdiction of the client's attempted solution—and we assume that when an intervention is successful, it is likely that one or more other suggestions and ways of promoting them could also have worked. The basic guideline, of course, is what tack do we want the client to abandon in favor of an alternative behavior that is more likely to be effective.

Q: Would you describe what was happening in treatment sessions 3 through 6, the period after the strategy was suggested and before the mother implemented it? What factors prevented this treatment from being even more efficient (i.e., requiring fewer sessions)?

A: Much of the time during those sessions was still spent with Bob in an attempt to develop more active participation despite our appraisal that he was not a complainant. It is probable that if we had not started with him, we would not have invested the further time as we did. In any case, since this was atypical, we do not feel that additional detail about our efforts with Bob would add to the reader's understanding of what we do, more typically, in our treatment approach. Obviously, if we had proceeded more as usual—started with the mother—we would have been able to save time. We probably would have seen her son only once and also had more continuity in monitoring her compliance with suggestions and their relative success. In any case, saving two or three sessions seems hardly consequential when so much treatment is still measured in terms of years.

Q: What is the average number of sessions that people are seen in treatment? How often do people come back for "booster sessions" after completing the original treatment?

A: Our average number of sessions in the Brief Therapy Center is about 6 1/2. When we see a case for less than our maximum of 10 sessions, we often, but not always, will tell the client that the remaining sessions are "in the bank," as we did in this case. This primarily is done as a measure of reassurance—you are not completely abandoned and on your own, you can call on us if need be. But given such reassurance, the need seems to arise very rarely.

Q: How long is your average treatment session? If people have 10 sessions in which to work, can these be divided into half or quarter sessions?

A: Our usual treatment session is one hour. We do not divide our sessions into smaller units, but from time to time we will stop a session short of the hour, with the patient's acquiescence, especially when we feel an important intervention has been made and we do not want to dilute it by further talk.

Q: How did you become a brief therapist?

Weakland: Not surprisingly, when colleagues discover that I began professional life as a chemical engineer, I am often asked, "How did you become a family therapist particularly interested in brief therapy?" This is not an easy question to answer briefly; only a few turning points can be mentioned.

I spent 6 years in research, development, and plant design as an engineer. I decided to get out of this field when, at last working for a highly competent and well-organized engineering firm, it became increasingly apparent to me that my daily work was like working on an assembly line—technical, but highly specialized and repetitive.

So I returned to graduate school to study sociology and anthropology; I had become interested in the social sciences and psychology through reading plus curiously observing behavior in the organizations in which I had been working. Several years later, I was invited by Gregory Bateson, my first teacher of anthropology, to work with him on some research on communication for which he had just received funding and I accepted.

This communication research covered a wide range, but after a while the work began to focus on studying the communication of schizophrenic patients in the Palo Alto VA Hospital where the project offices were located. Since we were always concerned with the context as well as the content of communication, it was only a next step to begin interviewing patients together with their family members. This, plus the influence of Don Jackson, who had joined us as a consultant on schizophrenia, led to attempts to do therapy with these families. This became one of the main origins of the whole family therapy movement.

At about the same time, Jay Haley and I became interested in hypnosis and began periodic visits to Phoenix to talk with Milton Erickson to discuss hypnosis and also his work with schizophrenic patients. During these meetings it became clear that Erickson often worked quite briefly, and that his work usually involved active behavioral intervention.

As I continued working in family therapy at MRI, which Jackson founded, I was pleased to see that family therapy was developing and spreading. I was not pleased, however, when I began to see articles appear with statements like, "After only a year of family therapy, the nature of the family's problem was becoming clear." After all, work with families had originally been seen (like psychoanalysis) as an effective, and therefore brief, approach to resolving problems, so when Richard Fisch proposed that a small group of us at MRI get together and experiment with keeping treatment brief by focusing on the main presenting problem and very active intervention, I was glad to join with him, and I have not regretted it over 20 some years.

In summation, my story is, "One thing leads to another."

Fisch: I would say it began; if there can be such a thing as a beginning, when I was an undergraduate, majoring in premed. I had the good fortune of taking a couple of classes in sociology from a creative and exciting instructor and I found it appealing to think of people's behavior in terms of social organization and culture. In choosing my psychiatric residency, I think this played a factor in selecting a Sullivanian institute rather than a strict Freudian one. However, much of the training was still Freudian and I recall feeling impatient at the mystification of the therapy process.

When I started working, mostly analytically, it became increasingly uncomfortable to spend much of my day sitting behind a couch while my patients talked into the air and I finally asked my patients if they would be more comfortable sitting up. That "simple" procedural change, of course, changes one's therapy; one is inclined to be more active. This, I think, contributed to a next step, a curiosity about husbands who set up appointments for their wives and accompany them to the appointment even though most of the wives were capable of driving.

My curiosity led me to ask the spouses if it would be all right if I saw them together. I was struck by the fact that in most cases, the husband seemed more discomfited by the wife's problem than his wife was. Without realizing it, this started putting me on the path of looking at things from an interactional rather than from an intrapsychic explanation. From this, I found myself taking another step by taking some training in family therapy at MRI. This was in 1960, and at that time, family therapy was a very new and exciting approach. At the same time, it gave me an opportunity to get to know some of the people at MRI. Among them was Jay Haley.

At that time, Haley had just written *Strategies of Psychotherapy* (Haley, 1963), and while I was intrigued by his ideas, I still regarded them as too superficial compared with the "real" and "deep" psychodynamic therapy I was still accustomed to using. However, one day I was presented with a patient who spoke almost no English and, in desperation, I mechanically applied the techniques Haley had used in an analogous case. The fact that it worked and quickly (a couple of weeks) put me another step away from my psychoanalytic background and on the path to a problem-solving approach. My therapy became a mélange of psychodynamic and family therapy, but when I got stuck, I resorted to a problem-oriented—"prescribing the symptom" approach, and enough of the time it got the therapy unstuck and the problem resolved. Without planning it, I began to use it more and more, even if I weren't stuck. Then I learned that Haley had gotten some of his inspiration from Milton Erickson and so, in the early 1960s, I took a couple of workshops with Erickson.

This interest in his work, plus the intrigue I found in the rapid changes that can occur in a case when approached in a problem-solving way, led to the next and probably most important step, the formation of the Brief Therapy Center in 1967, a project allowing me, John Weakland, Paul Watzlawick, and, later, many others to research more and more refined ways of shortening treatment and putting what we were doing into some comprehensive order. That was some 24 years ago, and I hope that I, we, continue to evolve into whatever paths it can take us.

# References

de Shazer, 5. (1985). *Keys to solution in brief therapy.* NY: W. W. Norton.

de Shazer, 5. (1988). Clues: Investigating solutions in brief therapy. NY: W.W. Norton.

Fisch, R., Weakland, J. H., & Segal, L. (1982). *The tactics of change: Doing therapy briefly.* San Francisco: Jossey-Bass.

Haley, J. (1963). *Strategies of psychotherapy.* NY: Grune & Stratton.

Watzlawick, P., Weakland, J. H., & Fisch, R. (1974). *Change: Principles of problem formation and problem resolution.* NY: W. W. Norton.

Weakland, J. H., Fisch, R., Watzlawick, R, & Bodin, A. H. (1974). Brief therapy: Focused problem resolution. *Family Process, 13,* 141-168.

# About the Editors

**Richard Fisch, M. D.,** is a psychiatrist who has been practicing in Palo Alto since 1958, after having completed a psychiatric residency at the Sheppard and Enoch Pratt Hospital, where Harry Stack Sullivan had done some of his earlier work. Among his educational experiences, Fisch values his years at the Bronx High School of Science in New York ("That's where I learned how to learn") and at Colby College in Maine, where he was greatly influenced by his instructor in anthropology, Dr. Kingsley Birge. Fisch received his medical training at the New York Medical College after a short sting at Columbia University School of Anthropology.

Introduced to family therapy through training he took in 1960 with Virginia Satir at the Mental Research Institute (MRI), Fisch became a research associate there in 1961, and later a senior research fellow. In 1965 Dr. Fisch proposed the creation of a research center focused specifically on making therapy more effective and efficient. Together with his colleagues at the institute, especially John Weakland and Paul Watzlawick, Fisch organized the Brief Therapy Center (BTC), and in early January 1967 began to see clients, which has continued uninterrupted to this day.

Dr. Fisch has four children living in disparate parts of the country: David in North Carolina, Amy in Los Angeles, Ben in Salinas and Sara, with husband Matt and baby Oliver, in San Francisco. For recreation, for years Fisch enjoyed flying as an instrument-rated pilot and he is seriously addicted to dark chocolate.

Recipient of awards for momentous contributions to Family Therapy and Brief Therapy from the American Family Therapy Association (AFTA) and the American Association for Marriage and Family Therapy (AAMFT), Dr. Fisch is co-author of the ground breaking books *Tactics of Change – Doing Therapy Briefly*, (with John H. Weakland and Lynn Segal), (1982); and *Change – Principles of Problem Formation and Problem Resolution*, (with Paul Watzlawick and John

Weakland), (1974); and more recently *Brief Therapy with Intimidating Cases* (with Karin Schlanger), (1999). In July 2007 Dr. Fisch retired both from private practice and from the MRI Brief Therapy Center. He now lives in quiet retirement in Menlo Park, California.

**Wendel A. Ray,** Ph.D., LCSW, LMFT, LPC, trained in Milan Systemic Family with Gianfranco Cecchin, and in clinical hypnosis at the M. H. Erickson Foundation. His doctoral studies were with Bradford Keeney in cybernetics applied to human behavior. Drawn to the Mental Research Institute (MRI) in 1987 to study the work of Don Jackson and the MRI Brief Therapy approach; he became an MRI Research Associate when John Weakland encouraged him to found the Don Jackson Archive. Dr. Ray has served as Teaching Faculty since that time, and as a member of the Brief Therapy Center from 1997–2004. MRI Director from 2000-2004, and a Senior Research Fellow, Dr. Ray continues to serve as Director of the Jackson Archive, a shared research project of MRI and The University of Louisiana at Monroe (ULM) Marriage and Family Therapy Program.

The Hammond Endowed Professor of Education (2008-2011) and Professor of Family System Theory in the Marriage and Family Therapy Doctoral and Master Degree Programs at ULM, Dr. Ray's research is in System, Cybernetic, and Communication Theory applied in understanding and changing human behavior. Dr. Ray teaches workshops and seminars across North and Central America, Europe, Africa, and Asia; and is author of more than 75 journal articles and book chapters. He is author or editor of a number of other books, a number of which have been published in several languages, including *Don D. Jackson: Interactional Theory in the Practice of Therapy, Selected Essays Volume II,* (Editor), (2009); *Paul Watzlawick: Insight May Cause Blindness and Other Essays* (Co-edited with Giorgio Nardone), (2009); *Don D. Jackson: Selected Essays at the Dawn of an Era, Volume 1,* (Editor), (2005); *Evolving Brief Therapies* (Co-edited with Steve de Shazer), (1998); *Propagations: 30 Years of influence from the MRI* (Co-edited with John Weakland), (1995); *Resource Focused Therapy* (Co-author with Brad Keeney), (1993); *The Cybernetics of Prejudices,* (1993), and *Irreverence,* (Co-author with Gianfranco Cecchin and Gerry Lane) (1992).

**Karin Schlanger, LMFT** is originally from Buenos Aires, Argentina. She studied clinical psychology and received her Licenciatura degree from the Universidad de Buenos Aires in 1982, where she first learned about the Mental Research Institute. She moved to Palo Alto following that dream in 1983. She immediately started working with Carlos Sluzki, then the director, and joined the Brief Therapy Center the following year. Mrs. Schlanger returned to school, receiving a degree in clinical psychology in 1987. She started her work with the

Latino population with Howard Liddle's group at San Francisco General Hospital, treating clients who were non-compliant with medical treatment. In 1997 she became the Assistant Director of the Brief Therapy Center and, since Dr. Fisch's retirement, in 2007 is Director of the BTC. She is a Senior Research Fellow at MRI since 1994, and author of numerous articles published internationally and, *Brief Therapy with Intimidating Cases* (1999) with Dr. Richard Fisch, which has been translated into five languages. Responding to the needs of low income, multiple problem, Latino clients and their families, she co-founded, with Barbara Anger-Díaz, the Latino Brief Therapy and Training Center. Since 1995, she has obtained numerous grants to work with the embattled public schools in East Palo Alto a high crime, low income community which is 75% Latino, 20% African American and 5% Pacific Islander. Since 2005 she has provided counseling and staff consultation for the East Palo Alto High School Academy, a public school created by Stanford University, School of Education to serve this population. Fluent in five languages—Spanish, English, French, Italian and German—Ms. Schlanger conducts training in MRI problem-solving Brief Therapy around the world as well as the United States. Karin is married to an agricultural engineer and has two sons, Felipe and Andreas.